A Rainbow Book

*A*pron *S*trings

Inheriting Courage,
Wisdom and ...
Breast Cancer

DIANE TROPEA GREENE

Rainbow Books, Inc.
FLORIDA

Library of Congress Cataloging-in-Publication Data

Greene, Diane Tropea, 1959–
    Apron strings : inheriting courage, wisdom, and breast cancer / by Diane
Tropea Greene. — 1st ed.
        p. cm.
    Includes bibliographical references.
    ISBN 1-56825-108-4 (trade softcover : alk. paper)
    1. Greene, Diane Tropea, 1959- 2. Breast—Cancer—Patients—Biography. 3. Breast—
Cancer—Patients—Family relationships. 4. Cancer—Genetic aspects. I. Title.
    RC280.B8G722 2007
    362.196'994490092—dc22
    [B]
                   2007008756

Apron Strings: Inheriting Courage, Wisdom and ...Breast Cancer © 2007 by Diane Tropea Greene

Author's Website: www.ApronStringsBook.com

ISBN-10: 1-56825-108-4 • ISBN-13: 978-1-56825-108-0

Published by

Rainbow Books, Inc., P. O. Box 430, Highland City, FL 33846-0430

Editorial Offices and Wholesale/Distributor Orders

Telephone: (863) 648-4420 • Email: RBIbooks@aol.com
www.RainbowBooksInc.com

Individuals' Orders

Toll-free Telephone (800) 431-1579 • www.AllBookStores.com

Disclaimer: The information contained in this publication is not intended as medical advice. Any use of the information in this publication is at the reader's discretion. The author and publisher specifically disclaim any and all liability arising directly or indirectly from the use or application of any information contained herein. A competent medical professional should be consulted regarding your specific situation.

Cover Photo: Courtesy of David A. Land
Author Photo © 2007 Christine Findlay / ChristineFindlayPhotoGraphicArts.com

The paper used in this publication meets the minimum requirements of the American National Standard for Information Sciences—Permanence of Paper for Printed Library Materials, ANSI Z39.48-1984.

First Edition 2007

13 12 11 10 09 08 07   7 6 5 4 3 2 1

Printed in the United States of America.

To my mom — Frances Tropea,
whose will and wisdom
continue to inspire me.

Special thanks to my sisters.
Though we've had our share of sorrow,
we still manage to enjoy life.

Pictured on the cover with the author (far right)
are her sisters, left to right:
Laura McGowan, Carol Wolkiewicz,
and Linda Phaneuf.

Contents

Part I:
Mom's Generation — A Threat Is Revealed

Part II:
My Generation — The Wisdom of Vigilance

$\mathcal{P}$reface

My reasons for writing this book are threefold.

First, it was written to honor the memory of friends and family who bravely faced their own cancers with courage, grace and dignity. I believe that everything happens for a reason, and although many of them sadly lost their battles, it is in large part because of them that I won mine. In a tragic twist of fate, had I not seen so much cancer in my early years, I am certain that I would not have been so diligent in my own screening.

Second, I feel that this book had to be written. Women (and men) need to know that there most certainly is life after breast cancer — even genetic breast cancer. So often I hear of women paralyzed with fear by the knowledge that they carry a mutation on one of the genes for breast cancer. Perhaps by reading the story of my family, they will come to realize, when facing adversity, that faith, love, humor and the strength of the human spirit will always prevail.

Finally, writing this book was a catharsis for me. From listening to my family's special memories of our departed loved ones, to delving back through my own journal entries from so long ago, this project filled me not only with hope but also with pride. The memory of all the special times spent with my family when my mother was alive, and the holidays with my aunts, uncles and cousins, put a smile on my face and brought joy to my heart. I am blessed to have grown up in a family with so much strength and tenacity.

My hope is that this book is read in the spirit in which it was written. Although at times it may cause a tear to be shed, it is not my intention to bring sadness. I would prefer that it be looked upon as a symbol of all that can be learned from the past — and all that the future has waiting for us. We only have to look for it.

Acknowledgments

There are so many people I wish to acknowledge who have helped me to be able to complete this labor of love.

First of all, to my family members who lost their battles with cancer: Bob Fraine, Frances Tropea, Nicky Fraine, Mary Jane Fraine, and Mary O'Connor - you are the inspiration not only for this book, but for my life. Your premature deaths were not in vain!

To my aunt, Francesca Fraine, and all of my cousins: thank you for graciously sharing your memories with me, so that I may better express at least some of the incredible fortitude with which our loved ones fought their battles.

To my dad, Peter Tropea, and my sisters–Linda Phaneuf, Laura McGowan and Carol Wolkiewicz: thank you for allowing me to share glimpses of our family life as we plodded through some very painful years. I am eternally grateful to you for permitting me to make public your own private struggles with genetic testing, so that others may benefit from your fearlessness.

I would like to express my gratitude to my cousin Patty Budka for consenting to share her experience, and becoming the first family member to prove that it is possible to be a breast cancer survivor.

Thank you to Bea Tusiani for encouraging me to write this book, and for helping me to believe that I actually could!

To the Adelphi NY Statewide Breast Cancer Hotline & Support Program, The Maurer Foundation for Breast Health Education, and Dr. Erna Busch-Devereaux, thank you for your support and endorsements. I would particularly like to express my gratitude to Dr. Busch-Devereaux for spending so much of your valuable time reading over my manuscript and giving me your medical expertise and references.

Thank you to Rita Samols for your wonderful editing, and to Jim Hall for your legal advice.

To my two beautiful sons, Matthew and Brian, thank you for never complaining when you arrived home from school to discover me with my head buried in the computer and dinner nowhere to be found. You are both, by far, my greatest joy. My wish is for all your days to be cancer-free and filled with love and laughter.

Lastly, to my husband and best friend, John (Jay) Greene, with whom all things are possible — I thank you for your unending love and support in this project, and in my life. You are my past, my present and my future. You will forever have my heart!

Part I

Mom's Generation – A Threat Is Revealed

September 1990

"Ninety-nine bottles of beer on the wall, ninety-nine bottles of beer ..."

Disrespectful — that's how it must have looked to anyone catching a glimpse of the school bus rolling up and down the cemetery lanes that crisp September afternoon.

"If one of those bottles should happen to fall .."

Anxious laughter echoed from inside as we chanted the familiar words of a childhood camp song, seemingly unaware of our surroundings.

"Ninety-eight bottles of beer on the wall!"

But we meant no disrespect. It was just that we had become all too familiar with the pain, anxiety, astonishment and sorrow of burying a loved one who succumbed to cancer. We were all too familiar with the ritual ... from diagnosis, to surgery, to treatments, to recurrence and, ultimately, to death. This was just our way of dealing with the pain.

I was cramped in my seat across from one cousin and behind another. My three sisters and six more cousins were scattered about, most of us under the age of 40. There were only two survivors from our parents' generation on the bus and the reality that we were fast becoming the "oldest generation" weighed heavily on our minds.

We had all been through this before. First it was Mom's brother — Uncle Bob. Next was Mom, then Uncle Nicky, and finally Aunt Mary Jane. All four siblings dying from the same disease: *cancer*. Three of them had *breast* cancer. Was it just a coincidence? Something in their neighborhood growing up? We didn't know. I'm not sure any of us really cared. We were just tired of the emotional and physical pain that cancer inflicts on a family. Those of us inside the bus knew far too well what it was like to lose a parent to cancer.

My dad was a school bus driver; unable to get the day off, he attended my aunt's burial service in the bus. Dad was at the wheel and Aunt Fran was there too, having lost her husband, Nicky, two years earlier. This was the fourth time in eight years that we had gathered together to bury a family member, none of them older than 60.

Aunt Mary Jane was buried in St. Raymond's Cemetery in the Bronx with the rest of her family. After the services we all climbed aboard Dad's bus to visit the graves of the rest of our departed relatives. The bus rambled up and down the rows of tombstones while we squinted to find the familiar names of the loved ones who had gone before us. Dad called out each name as we arrived at their resting places — *"Everyone off for Nicky... next stop: Bobby"* — as we clambered in and out of the bus at every stop.

As we realized that it looked more like a class trip than a solemn visit to hallowed grounds, the absurdity of the situation seemed to overtake us. In the midst of our collective grief, someone began singing "Ninety-nine Bottles of Beer on the Wall," and one by one the rest of us chimed in. When all else fails, and sadness and grief threaten to swallow you whole, what else can you do? Sing!

While counting down the fallen bottles, we went through the all-too-familiar burial ritual once more, this time masking our sorrow with song. It was a much-needed release, and knowing Aunt Mary Jane's good nature and silly sense of humor, she would have loved it.

In the Beginning

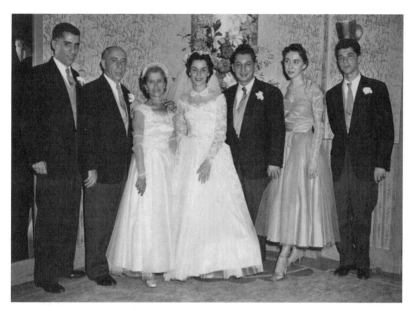

The Fraine Family. Mom and Dad's wedding: October 1954. Left to right: Uncle Bob, Grandpa, Grandma, Mom, Dad, Aunt Mary Jane, Uncle Nicky.

My mom and her family were from the Bronx, New York. She was the second of four children, two girls and two boys. Bob was the eldest; my mom, Frances, was next; then Mary Jane; and Nicky was the baby.

Dad was also from the Bronx. Shortly after he and Mom married, they moved into a two-family home owned by my mom's parents. Grandma and Grandpa lived upstairs along with Aunt Mary Jane, and Mom and Dad were in the apartment downstairs. All four of my parents' children were born in that house.

I am the third of four daughters born into our Italian Catholic family. Linda was the first, followed by Laura the next year. I was born three years later, and Carol rounded out the family five years after me.

Four daughters and eight breasts, born into a family which, decades later we would discover, carried a deadly gene mutation.

It was probably a blessing in disguise that Mom would not live long enough to realize that she and her siblings shared more than just the grave commonality of cancer. Long after their deaths, science would reveal the possibility that our family carried a genetic mutation that greatly increased the risk for breast and other cancers. Genetic carriers have a 50/50 chance of passing the mutant gene on to their children — the knowledge of which would have killed my mother before the cancer could. Although there is no definitive way of knowing if Mom or her siblings carried this mutation, their deaths and further investigation by my generation would reveal the strong possibility that they did.

Mom

The complex relationship between mother and daughter is magnified when it is cut short by sickness and death. At 23 years old I was no longer a child when Mom passed, but I was still living under my parents' roof and therefore abiding by their rules. I was expected to have dinner with the family at 6 o'clock every night and was still obliged to phone home if I was going to be out late. Both parents were very much authority figures in my life. Mom didn't live long enough for us to forge the woman-to-woman bond I so desperately coveted.

My mother held a tight rein on our family and was incredibly strong and opinionated. She had something to say about everything and everyone, usually believing she was right. At work, Mom felt that she could do things better than her coworkers and superiors, and she would often comment about how others dressed or the fact that they were lazy. She could be very cynical.

As a typical teenager, I often disagreed with her. I felt that she was judgmental and didn't always give others the benefit of the doubt. As I matured, however, I came to realize that what I once mistook as cynicism was often Mom's way of guiding her daughters. If she commented on someone's clothing, it was only because she felt that person was inappropriately dressed. And she was instilling a good work ethic when she didn't tolerate inefficiency in the office. My mother didn't gossip and was never hurtful. Her feelings were shared only with her family in her effort to impart her morals and values.

Mom had uncanny insight into others' psyches. Her first impression was often correct. Sometimes she'd infuriate me with a particularly harsh judgment of a friend or, worse yet, boyfriend; but almost without exception, Mom was right. Sharply perceptive, she could tell a lot about a person's character in only one or two encounters.

Money was very tight so my mother would often go without in order to buy one of us something we really wanted. With family as her first priority, she would do anything for us and wanted nothing more than to see her four little girls grow up to be honest, loving, productive women. Material possessions meant nothing to her. Once, when an acquaintance was bragging about her jewels, Mom quipped, "I have four gems of my own at home. They are called Linda, Laura, Diane and Carol."

When it came to education, both Mom and Dad felt that if you didn't know exactly what profession you wanted to enter you were just wasting your time going to college. They believed that we would be better off going directly into the working world, that on-the-job training was better than any degree, and that we would probably all marry and have children anyway, leaving careers behind. Just goes to show how times have changed!

Being somewhat confused and obedient, I followed their advice and went straight to work after high school, eventually going back to college when I was well into my 30s. Knowing that my parents acted out of love and in our best interests, I don't fault them for my choice. By the time I went to college I already had a solid work background, and was mature enough to realize that it was a privilege, not an obligation,

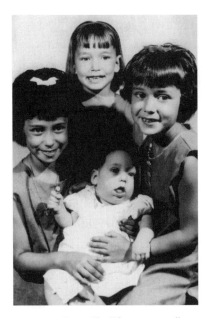

Mom and Dad's "four gems" — **1964.** Left to right: Linda, Me (top center), Laura, Carol (on lap).

to continue my education. So it all worked out for the best.

Mothering four girls had its joys and sorrows. There were the inevitable fights over hogging the bathroom and borrowing one another's clothes, but as we got older the fighting stopped and friendships developed. Ours was the house that everyone "on the block" considered crazy. We would sing while cleaning up after dinner at night, sometimes even performing the songs from *Grease*. Our basement or front stoop was usually filled with our friends who thought that Mom and Dad were "cool." My family wasn't perfect, but I consider myself blessed to be a part of it.

$\mathcal{D}$ad

As a young man, my dad was the typical "tough guy" from the Bronx. He grew up in a neighborhood where fists were used to settle conflicts. Mom often joked that most of his friends were either dead or in jail.

When my father was 15 years old, his dad died of a heart attack. Becoming the man of the house at such a tender age, he reluctantly quit school so he could work to support his mother and younger sister.

Because his first love was boxing, Dad became a professional fighter. At only 5 feet 6 inches tall, he was nicknamed "Little Pete." Much of his youth was spent at the gym hanging out with the guys. Unfortunately, boxing didn't pay the bills, so Dad gave it up as a profession and took on other jobs. He continued to keep his hand in boxing for years to come, but chose to train fighters instead of entering the ring himself.

Dad was something of a jack of all trades. As a very young man he worked at just about any job he could find, whether it was plumbing, electrical work or even auto mechanics. He finally settled on a job as a milkman, the first occupation from which he would retire.

After marrying in 1954, Mom and Dad continued to live in my grandparents' house while longing for one of their own. Over a decade later, with four daughters in tow, Dad had finally saved enough money to move his family of six into our very own home in Queens. Shortly thereafter, my grandparents left the Bronx and moved, along with Aunt Mary Jane, onto the very next block.

Thrilled to finally be living the American dream, Dad had to hustle to make ends meet. He worked on the milk route from the wee hours of the morning until late afternoon, and then was off to tend bar well past midnight, only to repeat the cycle the next day. Believing his wife should stay at home while their children were young, Dad would often take on odd jobs to make a little extra cash. He sold plants and paintings at a roadside gas station and even did home repairs for one of the neighbors, managing to make a good life for his family despite his humble beginnings.

As a child I remember being embarrassed by my dad's occupation. While most of my friends' parents were blue collar workers as well, few had to take on odd jobs to supplement their incomes. We were the only family in the neighborhood that seldom took vacations or went out to dinner. I wore a lot of hand-me-downs from my sisters and cousins, and always wound up with a secondhand bicycle. My parents drove a used car, frequently in disrepair. I was constantly afraid that my friends were going to think we were poor.

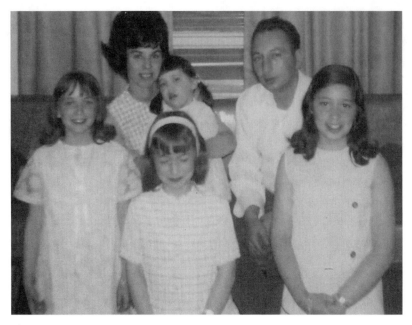

Our Family — 1966. Left to right: Laura, Mom, Carol (in arms), Dad, Me (headband), Linda.

As for parenting, Dad left most of that to my mom. I don't believe it was lack of interest; I think he just didn't know how to relate to four daughters. He desperately wanted a son with whom he could share his interests. He would jokingly introduce us as Louie, Larry, Danny and Carl when we were young and accompanied him to his bowling league or the Golden Gloves boxing matches. That novelty ended as our interests turned to clothes, boys and makeup when we entered our teens.

But there was still hope. When we began bringing boyfriends home, Dad was delighted to finally have some male comrades. After being challenged to paddle-ball matches and defeated in push-up competitions, our poor unsuspecting dates would be roped into helping him install an air conditioner or fix a leaky roof. Although my sisters and I were embarrassed by his antics, the guys usually were happy to help him out because Dad was really fun to be around.

A fairly easygoing man, he wasn't perturbed by the nonsense that consumes young girls, and would remain unscathed by the door-slamming, name-calling and other estrogen-related drama in our household. But when the mood turned to more important issues — like staying out past curfew or talking back to him — heads would roll. On those occasions you could almost see the blood boiling under his skin as he tried to restrain himself from striking us. That was, after all, the way Dad had solved his own conflicts as a child.

Living with five women, he would often complain that we were all against him. Truth be told, we did pick on him, especially since he wasn't exactly the classiest guy around. My father would think nothing of belching or blowing his nose right at the dinner table. On holidays he would lie down in the middle of a house full of company and take a nap amid the hustle and bustle. This would infuriate my mother, and the rest of us would chime right in. But what he lacked in class he more than made up for in character.

I've rarely heard my father say a bad word about anyone; whether a janitor or the CEO of a company, Dad treats them exactly the same. My father never sees anyone as black, white, Irish, Jewish, etc. He sees just the person, not ethnicity. Both of my parents instilled in us a respect for others as equals.

Looking back and realizing that wealth has little to do with income, we were probably the richest family I know. How ungrateful I was to have been embarrassed by the fact that my parents worked several jobs to ensure our stability! I grew up in a home where there was a very strong work ethic and we were welcome to bring our friends over anytime we wanted. A home where we ate dinner together every night and my parents always knew where we were and who we were with. The kind of home I hope I am providing today for my own children.

Growing Up Italian

The decor in many Italian-American homes during the 60s and 70s was unlike that of any other ethnic group, and ours was no exception. Our living room was furnished entirely in Italian Provincial, complete with crushed-velvet sofa and chairs, wall-to-wall draperies fastened with rope-tassel tiebacks, and an oversized velvet-backed oil painting of a horse-drawn chariot. Mirrors, gold and cherubs abounded and all the furniture was protected by plastic slipcovers!

My grandfather contributed to this highly stylized décor. Working in the packing department of a hand blown-glass factory, he rescued all the damaged figurines from the garbage pile and, like a surgeon, pieced together their broken bodies on a makeshift operating table set up in his basement. Grandpa was quite proud of his surgical prowess and would pass these newly reborn statues on to his children. Therefore, in addition to all the gaudy gold and velvet, my entire extended family had numerous glass collectibles on display, each in various stages of distress. One might be missing a hand or a foot, while another might have had his head glued back on. The one I remember most vividly was Don Quixote, minus a foot, displayed front and center in my grandparents' living room bay window. I don't know why it never occurred to me that my family's home was different in this respect from the homes of everyone else I knew. I suppose it could be attributed to the innocence of childhood.

Holidays at an Italian home are unique as well. The meal was the center of everything, and once you sat down at the table there was no turning back. Each dining experience consisted of at least four courses: antipasto, soup, macaroni and, finally, meat with all the trimmings. Dinner would end with coffee — brown or black — brown being regular coffee and black being espresso, served with anisette. Pastries or Italian cheesecake usually rounded out the meal along with plentiful bowls of nuts and fruit.

My grandparents and Aunt Mary Jane were always on hand during the holidays, as they were an important part of my early years. In addition to the holiday feasts, every Sunday morning we would get together for breakfast. After mass Grandpa would scoot off to the bakery to buy our favorite "buns and rolls" and we would all enjoy sharing our morning meal. Often we would get together again on Sunday evening for coffee and cake. While I didn't realize it at the time, this was a tradition I would come to treasure.

Uncle Bob

"I'll ask Bobby." That's what I remember about Uncle Bob. Whenever my mother had a question that required an educated answer, she'd call her brother Bob.

He was the only member of my mom's family with a college degree. My mom was a high school graduate, as was her sister, Mary Jane, and brother Nicky. Only Uncle Bob had completed college, and it was he who everyone called with questions about legal matters, finances or taxes.

Mom really looked up to her older brother, ten years her senior. He was tall and very handsome. Uncle Bob lived with his family in Rockland County, New York. To those of us who still lived in the boroughs, this was considered "the country." He was married to Mary, and they had five children — Bobby, Terry, Patty, John and Mary.

Uncle Bob was the first to get cancer. He had breast cancer. It was the 1970s, and I had never heard of a man getting breast cancer. I remember seeing him bare-chested and it looked so strange to see one whole side sunken in, without a nipple. Unlike a woman, it's very hard for a man to conceal a mastectomy, since there is no bra in which to hide a prosthesis.

I was in my early teens when Uncle Bob first got sick. I remember hearing all the terms — malignant, benign, chemotherapy, radiation. We discussed these things around the dinner table when I was growing

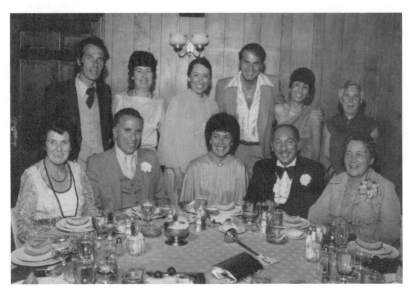

Mom and Dad's Table at Laura and Jim's Wedding. Top left to right: Uncle Nicky, Aunt Fran, Aunt Mary Jane, Uncle Tommy (Dad's brother-in-law), Aunt Marie (Dad's sister), Madeline (Dad's Godmother). Bottom left to right: Aunt Mary, Uncle Bob, Mom, Dad, Grandma (Dad's Mom).

up. It was all rather matter-of-fact to me; I didn't realize at the time how strange the dinner conversation was.

Little by little, Uncle Bob got sicker. It started with his breast when he was 51. The cancer spread to multiple organs including his prostate and testicles. He died in 1982 and was buried on his 60th birthday. Though he was the first one to die of the disease, it would turn out that he would be the eldest at his death.

Journal Entry — Tuesday, January 26, 1982
When I got home tonight, I found out that Uncle Bob died. Dad, Linda and Laura went to see him this past Sunday and everyone was talking about how bad he looked. I have mixed feelings ... what is life really worth and why are we even here? It is all so weird. I just hope and pray his family can handle it.

We were unaware that my uncle's funeral service was just the beginning of the sorrow that would ensue. Thankfully, we all had a sense of humor. You see, prior to meeting and marrying my Aunt Mary, Uncle Bob had explored the possibility of a life in the seminary, thus he still had many priest friends. There must have been ten priests officiating at his funeral. After the blessing of the bread and wine, when all the priests placed the host in their mouths and began to chew, it seemed as if the whole church echoed with munching sounds! As I desperately struggled to stifle my own nervous giggle, I spotted Aunt Mary with all five of their children in the first pew. One by one you could see their shoulders bobbing up and down as everyone finally allowed a little laughter to lessen their sorrow. This would be the first of many times that humor would help us to cope.

At the time of my uncle's death, my mother was fighting a battle of her own. Several years earlier she, too, had been diagnosed with breast cancer, and by 1982 she was too sick to attend her own brother's funeral.

Mom's Diagnosis

I was 17 when my mother was diagnosed with cancer. It was the summer of 1977 and I was in a three-week training class for my first full-time job. My mother was having surgery to remove a lump in her breast. Back then the decision to remove either just the tumor or the entire breast was made during the operation, so it was a shock when she awoke to find that her doctor had removed the cancerous breast in a procedure called a total mastectomy.

I remember being called out of my training class to take the phone call from my sister Linda advising me of Mom's mastectomy. I was very upset, but at the time my uncle had been fighting and apparently winning his battle with breast cancer, so I just assumed that Mom would do the same. I suppose I was still under the childish assumption that things like that happened only to "other people." I would soon be proven wrong.

Journal Entry — Thursday, August 18, 1977
Linda called me at work to tell me Mom's tumor is cancerous and that she had her breast removed. I cried at first, but they feel they "got it all" so that's a big relief ...

We visited Mom in the hospital on the first night after her surgery. She was groggy from the medication and was lying in bed softly moaning. A tube, where her breast had been, drained the excess fluid and blood from the surgical site until the tissues would begin to heal. I remember feeling so helpless. It all seemed so cruel. Dad was speechless, not knowing what to say or do. I felt as if life as I once knew it was now over. I sensed that things would never be the same.

...Saw Mom tonight. She was unconscious and in a lot of pain. It was upsetting me a lot to see her like that. Dad had tears in his eyes. I hope she feels better tomorrow.

To my astonishment, the very next day we visited Mom and she was sitting up in bed, hair done and makeup on! We were all so relieved. Things were going to be okay after all. That was the first of many times that within her own despair, Mom found the inner strength to pull herself together for her family. She came home after a few days, and all was right with the world.

Since reconstructive surgery was not widely used at the time, my mother pinned a prosthesis into her bra, which she would hang over the bathroom doorknob at night. She showed us her scar to alleviate any curiosity and fear of the unknown, and was very open about the whole situation. Living with so much cancer around me was becoming rather commonplace.

Although breast cancer was still quite a taboo subject, when Mom returned to work she knew her co-workers would be uncomfortable and curious. So, right from the start she told them to take a good look at her chest and get it over with, instead of milling about not knowing where to focus their eyes.

For several years after her initial diagnosis, life went on normally. My sisters and I even managed to scrape together enough money to send my parents to Europe for their 25th wedding anniversary. Laura married and bought her first house. Carol graduated from high school and started college. Linda became engaged, and I began taking college courses at night. Life was moving predictably forward and we were starting to feel that Mom was going to beat

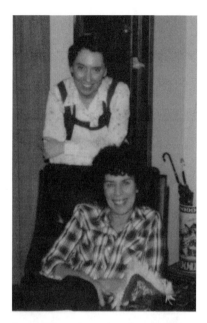

Aunt Mary Jane (top) and Mom. In 1981.

her cancer, even though her brother had now taken a step backward in his battle. But just weeks before my Uncle Bob's death, Mom was diagnosed with lung cancer.

Journal Entry — Monday, January 4, 1982

What a terrible nightmare! Mom had surgery this morning and they said it is cancer and there is not much they can do. I feel so helpless and depressed. I am so afraid for her. I am really going to need strength. It's certainly going to be a bad year. All we can do is hope and pray. I can accept death, but I will not be able to accept her being in any pain. It's just not fair. She is much too good a person. Dad is holding up pretty well, but you can see the pain in his eyes.

Ironically, Mom's breast cancer had not metastasized (spread) to her lungs. This was a new cancer, a direct result of her years of cigarette smoking. How maddening that Mom actually survived her *breast* cancer, a disease she had no control over, only to die from lung cancer, a disease she quite possibly could have avoided had she not been such a heavy smoker! Now her battle was intensifying.

Several surgeries followed, as well as the requisite radiation and chemotherapy. She lost all her hair from the chemo and had permanent scars from the radiation burns, but she continued to keep a positive, upbeat attitude and even found some humor in it all. Once, upon being presented with a huge doctor's bill, Mom joked, "I think there's been a mistake here. I don't want to buy the building, I just want to pay the bill." Her optimism and wit inspired those around her, including me.

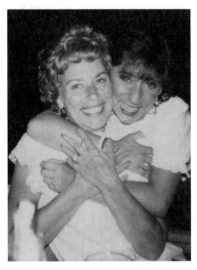

Carol with Mom. In her blonde wig in 1982.

My mother continued to work throughout all her treatments. Although her hair loss was devastating, she had some fun with her wigs, even buying a blonde one as a change from her naturally jet-black hair.

The ensuing months would bring many changes. There were treatments and occasional surgeries and hospital stays, but she plugged along as best as she could. Though we were all aware that the cancer was spreading, somehow we still managed to live for the moment, right up until that horrible day when the doctors told her they had exhausted all their resources and there was nothing more they could do for her. Mom was told that she was terminally ill. Many people in her predicament would simply wait to die, but not my mother. There was no way she was going to just sit around waiting to die!

Our family talked for hours that night. There were so many things Mom wanted to say, but it was hard for her to put her feelings into words. She felt that she "wasn't done yet," and she struggled to find some "profound words" to leave us, words we could draw strength from for the rest of our lives.

She asked us to be patient with Dad and accept anyone he might meet in the future. Mom knew that my dad was the type of man who needed a woman around, and she wanted to be sure that we would understand. Even facing death, my mother was more concerned about her family than she was about herself.

Journal Entry — Tuesday, October 19, 1982

Well, our worst fears have been confirmed. The doctor discovered that the cancer spread to Mom's head and hip. Now she is terminal. We all sat around crying and laughing and crying again, and discussing how we feel and telling Mom that we love her. She was saying she had so much she wanted to say but didn't know how to say it. It certainly was a dramatic, heart-wrenching scene. Sometimes I feel strong and other times I just want to die along with her.

In November 1982 Mom became immobilized after tripping over a chair at work, and could barely walk. No longer able to climb the stairs to bed, she began sleeping on the living room couch, while Dad slumbered on the floor beside her. He installed a telephone in the living room and Mom built her shrinking world around the sofa where she sat, slept and even ate her meals. The room was transformed into a mini–hospital ward, with her walker, wheelchair and medications surrounding her.

Laura had married a few years earlier and now it was Linda's turn. As the wedding rapidly approached and Mom got sicker, she decided to fill her idle days with something productive. She made a bridal doll dressed in an exact replica of Linda's wedding gown, as well as four bridesmaid dolls as her attendants, to be displayed at Linda's bridal shower.

That wasn't enough for my time-conscious mother. Still struggling with the notion of leaving behind something for all of us to cherish, she proceeded to hand-stitch a magnificent white satin christening outfit along with a crocheted sweater set for the grandchildren she so desperately wanted but would never meet. All ten grandchildren were christened in the gown Mom made, and her legacy lives on in each and every grandchild.

Christmas was bittersweet that year. Mom was confined to a wheelchair and her body was swollen from the steroid medications. She had trouble breathing and sometimes had to rely on an oxygen tank. We knew the end was near.

On a late night in February Mom's breathing became increasingly labored and we could no longer keep her comfortable. She argued that she didn't want to go into the hospital, knowing she would never return home, but we didn't have a choice. In the middle of the night she and Dad got into the ambulance for a trip to the hospital from where, as Mom predicted, she would never return.

She remained there several days. The night before her death, our whole family gathered at her bedside. Mom had the vacant stare that I have come to recognize as the "death look." Her eyes were wide open but didn't appear to focus on anything. She was so drugged with morphine that she slipped in and out of lucidity. I will never forget kissing her goodbye for the last time. She looked at us and said, "You're all leaving me now?" *No, Mom, it's you who is leaving us.* I kissed her goodbye and whispered, "I love you." I'd always had a hard time saying that to her, but this time it was easy. The rest of us went home, but Dad spent the night. It was February 13, 1983, and a big snowstorm was forecast.

Journal Entry — Sunday, February 13, 1983

My head is pounding, my stomach is in a knot and I feel like throwing up. We all went to see Mom today. She is in pain — all drugged up and doesn't know what's going on. I can't stop crying. I cannot believe that the woman who gave birth to me is dying. My mother is dying.

I tossed, turned and cried all night. I just couldn't believe that this was happening. I knew that cancer was going to kill my mother; I just didn't think it was going to be *now*. When the phone rang in the early morning hours, the first thought that passed into my head was *Thank*

God, it's over. Linda picked it up and I heard her say, "She's gone?" It was Valentine's Day, and overnight more than a foot of snow had fallen.

Journal Entry — Monday, February 14, 1983
Mom died at 6:15 this morning. Dad was with her. I can hardly believe it. My hand is writing this, but my heart doesn't believe I will not ever see my mother again. My mother is gone. But she will always be a part of what I do and who I am, and that will never go away. I think Mom knows that. Can she see me now?

It would be 17 years before I learned that I had inherited not only a deadly genetic predisposition from Mom, but also the strength and courage I would need to face that reality. Ultimately, the most profound legacy my mother left behind was her *desire* to leave us with just that ... something profound.

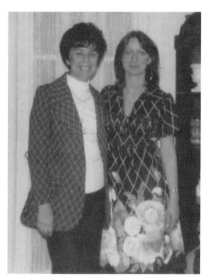

One of the Few Pictures of Mom and Me. On my high school graduation day in 1977.

Moving Forward After Mom's Death

While my mother's life was coming to an end, mine was just beginning. I had found love in, of all places, the house next door! Jay literally lived next door to my family, with our homes even sharing a common driveway. He had been my best friend and confidant for years. As our friendship began turning into love during the months my mother was sick, it was Mom who opened my eyes to it. I was too afraid to lose my best friend if our new love didn't work out, but Mom eloquently advised me to "crap or get off the pot." I took her advice and found that true love and friendship go hand in hand. We started dating right before my mother passed away, and I cannot imagine how I would have faced the next year without Jay's unending love and support.

Journal Entry — Monday, February 21, 1983
I am already having trouble controlling my emotions. Cleaned out Mom's closet and that was a relief. The four of us sisters started talking and crying and arguing. We seem to have worked it all out and now I feel 100 percent better. Went to the park with Jay and we walked and talked and it felt great. I love him incredibly. I never would have made it without him. I love him so much! I wonder if Mom knew our relationship was inevitable.

For several months after Mom died we sisters all did our best to get along. Linda took on the role of "homemaker," coordinating most of the cleaning, cooking and laundry. Her wedding was just three months away, and Dad was getting increasingly nervous about her moving out. Carol and I did our part as well, but he believed that when Linda left things would never run as smoothly. I suppose because she was his eldest daughter, he had the most confidence in her. Three months to the day after Mom's death, Linda and Al married. Now it was just Dad and his two youngest, Carol and me.

Life got pretty tough after that. Dad expected everything to run as smoothly as when Mom was still alive. Carol was in college and I was working full time and taking courses several nights a week, so it was a juggling act to maintain the household. In the evenings and on weekends she and I did our best to make up for it, but we never seemed to meet Dad's expectations. Sometimes I'd spend hours cleaning or cooking only to have him berate me because it wasn't exactly the way Mom would have done it.

Although Linda and Laura tried their best to sympathize, there wasn't really any way they could know just how overwhelmed Carol and I were. It was a really emotional time, and we often felt as if it was us against the rest of the world! It was almost impossible to remember that our home had once was been the "place to be," alive with activity and laughter. My family, as I had known it, would never again be the same.

What I failed to realize at the time was that while I was mourning my mother's death and the loss of the family circle I was accustomed to, I still had a person in my life with whom I planned to grow old. Dad had been robbed of the many wonderful years he might have had with my mother. As I rapidly approach my parents' age at Mom's death, I am finally beginning to understand the magnitude of my father's loss. How many conflicts could be averted if we were born with the wisdom that time and experience affords us?

At the time of my mother's death, the torch had already been passed to her brother Nicky, the third sibling diagnosed with cancer.

Uncle Nicky

Nicky was the youngest of Mom's siblings and, rumor has it, the mischievous one. I never tire of the stories repeated over and over again about his many childhood high jinks.

Nicky owned a gas station in his hometown of Rye, New York, where he lived with his wife, Fran, and their three daughters — Michele, Renee and Carla. As with Mom's other siblings, we spent many holidays as a family unit. Uncle Nicky always had a funny story to tell about their childhood years in the Bronx.

I can remember the glint in his eye as he good-naturedly teased my mother about the time he got his arm stuck in the agitator of the washing machine while on her watch. Mom would retaliate by showing everyone her knee, still bearing a faint trace of lead from the pencil he stabbed her with during a childhood argument. Uncle Nicky and his family were fun to be around, and my sisters and I always enjoyed spending time with them.

In 1983, toward the end of my mother's life, Nicky was diagnosed with cancer. Unlike the others, my uncle's cancer did not start in his breast. His was a very uncommon form of cancer known as adenoid cystic carcinoma, which started in his head. Sadly, it progressed in much the same way as it did in Uncle Bob and my mom. Eventually, Nicky's cancer spread to his neck, eye, and bones. And much like his brother and sister before him, my uncle approached his cancer with the utmost class and dignity, and sometimes even a little humor.

At one point in his journey, a tumor behind his eye needed surgery. My uncle opted to be awake for this innovative procedure in which a radioactive disk was inserted behind the cornea. As his eye was being manipulated into different positions, my uncle joked with the nurses that he could see down their blouses and up their skirts! The doctors told my aunt that they seldom witness such a great sense of humor under such dire circumstances.

When radiation was required, Nicky was apprehensive that the rays might be targeting his eye, or even his brain, instead of the tumor. On one occasion, when he expressed concern to the nurse who was prepping him, she pooh-poohed his unease. Begrudgingly, my uncle complied and allowed her to wheel him into the lab for the thirty-second zap of radiation. When that same nurse wheeled him back out afterward she commented condescendingly, "There, now, that wasn't so bad, was it?" My uncle replied with an incoherent "Blub blobby boo doo poo."

She proceeded to scream "Code blue, code blue! Dr. Smith, get in here STAT!" Hospital workers came running, all barking commands and asking him questions, which he ignored. Finally the doctor came in and asked, "Nick, Nick, can you hear me? What day is it? Do you know where you are?"

My uncle answered the doctor correctly and without hesitation, to which the doctor replied, "What happened in here?" Nicky shrugged and with a look of total innocence smirked, "I have no idea. One minute the nurse is wheeling me back from my treatment, and the next she's screaming and yelling down the hall like a lunatic." At that point the nurse practically lunged at him while shouting obscenities. The doctor had to turn his back on both of them to hide his amusement.

Laughter heals the soul, but not always the body. As the cancer spread, Uncle Nicky's body began to deteriorate. When the cancer invaded his bones, it was strongly suggested that Nicky use marijuana to ease his intense pain. He wouldn't hear of it. My uncle absolutely refused to bring any drugs into the house with his three daughters there. His integrity remained strong.

In the end, Nicky was confined to a hospital bed in his home. When his youngest daughter, Carla, graduated from high school, my uncle insisted they have a backyard party for her, since they had done so for their other daughters. He spent most of the party on the front porch, in obvious pain, while friends and family gathered around him to spend some time.

At the end of the summer of 1988, Nicky was admitted to the hospital for the last time. During his hospital stay he experienced something quite extraordinary — something that would eventually bring peace to his wife, Fran, and their daughters. Across the street from the hospital was a supermarket with a sensor light on the wall — the type that lights up as darkness approaches. This particular weekend was bright and sunny and, despite his pain, my uncle was quite lucid — even speaking by phone to his youngest daughter, who was away at college.

His wife was at his bedside when he exclaimed, "Jesus is coming, look at the light across the way." My aunt looked out the window and the sensor light turned on. He then started to recite the Our Father. A minute or so later he said, "Jesus is leaving," and sure enough, the light went off. Mind you, my uncle's bed was too low to allow him to see out the window. Later that same afternoon it happened again. The following day Nicky asked to have his bed moved closer to the window so he could actually see the light himself.

Nicky died at the hospital on Labor Day Weekend, two days after "seeing the light." He was 51 years old. Unfortunately, it would be years before my aunt would be able to realize the full impact of my uncle's "light" episodes. It wasn't until speaking with a Jesuit priest years later that Fran was able to understand its significance. The cleric told her that God allowed Nicky to see Him prior to calling my uncle to His side, and that not everyone facing death is that fortunate. Although she longed to have many more years with her husband, my aunt was finally able to find some peace in that comforting thought.

Journal Entry — Sunday, September 18, 1988

Once again, some very sad things have happened. Uncle Nicky died. I really feel so bad. Everyone there seems to be doing extremely well. It's not as if they didn't know it was going to happen! Aunt Mary Jane is doing pretty well …Sometimes she amazes me. She's the only one left and must really be distraught, but she seems OK.

At the time of my uncle's death, his last surviving sister, Mary Jane, had already been diagnosed with cancer.

Aunt Mary Jane

Every young girl should have an Aunt Mary Jane in her life. She made everything fun. Never having married and with no children, she treated all her nieces and nephews as her own. I always felt that my sisters and I were the luckiest of all our cousins since Aunt Mary Jane lived right upstairs from us in the Bronx, and then on the very next block in Queens. We could see her anytime we wanted.

Aunt Mary Jane had several nicknames. As children, my sisters and I jokingly began calling her "Aunt Motza Ball," which was eventually shortened to "Motz." This name stayed with her to her death. Dad, on the other hand, preferred calling her "Tarzan," as in "Me Tarzan, You (Mary) Jane." Sometimes he shortened it further and just called her "Tarz." I suppose it wasn't any sillier than Aunt Motza Ball! Anyway, she took it all in stride even when Dad was teasing her. Make no mistake; we all loved Motz — even Dad. It's just that she was always — how can I put it gently — flaky. Once, upon being told by her gynecologist that she had a yeast infection, my aunt exclaimed, "But I don't even bake!"

Motz was the only person I ever knew who took the road test for her driver's license seven times. Yes, seven. When giving people directions to her house, she'd tell them to "get off at exit 17 and immediately get over to the right. Don't worry about everyone beeping at you, that's what they do at that exit." We all used to have such a chuckle over that. It really was a wonder that she never killed herself or someone else when she was behind the wheel.

My father always made fun of my aunt's lack of culinary skills. He'd swear that "Tarz can't even make a decent cup of coffee." I never understood how she could or why she would tolerate it, but being her good-natured self, she'd just laugh it off. I, on the other hand, couldn't have cared less about how well she could cook. Being at her house was always an adventure, and that's all that mattered to me.

Aunt Mary Jane worked in Manhattan as a secretary. She always had the nicest clothes and jewelry. Sometimes when we were visiting, she'd let us go into her dresser drawers and jewelry box. We'd always come away from one of our visits with a bagful of goodies — maybe an admired pin, a pair of earrings or a hair clip. She just loved to give things to us. Occasionally, she would even take us to work with her. That was the best! We would ride the subway and go out to lunch. I always treasured those special days.

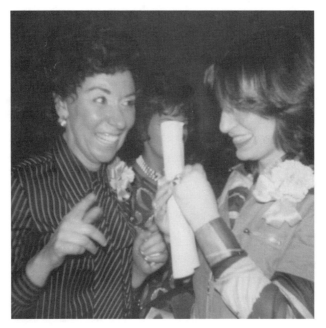

Motz. Presenting me with my class ring — 1976.

When I received my class ring in high school, it was Motz I invited to the Ring Day Ceremony — indeed, a very special honor at my all-girl Catholic high school. She took the whole day off from work to share in my joy and present me with my ring.

After graduating with a secretarial degree, I got my first job in Manhattan. Motz worked nearby and we would often go to lunch together. Acutely aware of my limited finances, she occasionally would treat me despite my protests. I always felt bad that she had to dip into her own wallet, but secretly was relieved that she did so.

After both my grandparents passed away, Aunt Mary Jane bought a place of her own. She was 48 years old. Luckily, her co-op apartment was only a twenty minute drive from my house, so we continued to see her often. Our relationship grew as I matured. While she and my mom were completely different people, it was still comforting and reassuring to have Motz around after Mom died. Unfortunately, for her it wasn't as simple.

With her parents and all of her siblings gone, Motz was living by herself for the first time in her life. Though she was still very active, there were times, she confessed, when the loneliness overtook her and she would cry herself to sleep.

Before her seemingly inevitable diagnosis, Aunt Mary Jane had several benign lumps removed. She was 50 years old when she was informed that her luck had run out. My mom had been gone for two years. *Here we go again.*

When my aunt had her mastectomy, my sisters and I were all at the hospital. I remember the doctor coming out to tell us "We think we got it all," an expression I had come to know and detest. What exactly does that mean, "We think we got it all?" How about if we said "We think we'll pay your fee?" How confident does that make *you* feel? In any case, Motz recovered surprisingly well from her surgery and was back to work in no time. After a few years, as I had come to expect from past experience, her cancer began to metastasize.

Journal Entry — Tuesday, September 12, 1989

Aunt Mary Jane's cancer spread. She has four tumors in her brain and has to go for radiation. I have been so upset all week. She's been having blurred vision and dizziness for about two weeks. At first they told her it was an inner ear infection, but as usual, they found it to be cancer. She is beginning to act almost senile now. I think it's a combination of the tumors and her distraught state. We can only pray that she has minimal pain.

The next year, Aunt Mary Jane lost her battle. She was 55 years old.

Journal Entry — Monday, September 10, 1990
I am literally sitting here waiting for the phone call saying Aunt Mary Jane died.
She's running 106 fever, and her blood pressure is low. I should really be there but
Matthew is sick and I don't want to leave him with a sitter. She shouldn't have
to have a lonely death!

For as long as I live I will never forget the night of Aunt Mary Jane's death. She had been very ill for several months. We had arranged for her to have around-the-clock nursing care in her home. The nurses told us that the time was near, so we weren't surprised when the call came to say our good-byes. In my haste to arrange child care I was unaware that she had already passed away when I picked up my sister. Laura got in the car and started going into detail about my aunt's will and the funeral arrangements. I turned to her and said, "She *already died?*"

"I'm sorry, I thought you knew," she replied.

Sobs wracked my body and I had to pull over. After a moment or two I pulled myself together and we continued on our drive to bid farewell to our beloved aunt. The events that would unfold once we arrived were so surreal they became almost comical.

The moment we pulled into the parking lot I noticed that her apartment on the third floor looked eerily different than in the past. All the shades were up, with the lights and ceiling fan on in her bedroom. Aunt Mary Jane would never leave her shades up at a moment like this, I thought. It looked cavernous, cold and uninviting — as if when the life went out of her body, it also went out of her home.

In unspeakable grief, Laura and I got into the elevator, where we were joined by two EMS workers eager to save the life of the stranger on the third floor. Linda had already arrived; Carol, who lived in New Jersey, was unable to come.

Once inside, the EMS workers went about their task of trying to revive her. Aunt Mary Jane had a "do not resuscitate" (DNR) order. Why were they reviving her? We were all yelling for them to stop; why should they revive her now, so that she can die tomorrow? It didn't make any sense. But they wouldn't stop, even after we presented the signed DNR stating her intentions that no extraordinary measures be taken to revive her.

Having previously been instructed by my aunt's doctor, when Aunt Mary Jane stopped breathing, Linda dialed 911. She informed them that Motz was a terminal patient expected to die at home. We were told they would respect that wish when they arrived. Sadly, that wasn't the case. It was their job, they told us, to try to resuscitate her.

We were alternately begging them to stop and sobbing. Neighbors were ringing the bell to see if they could help. Emotions were high. It was a circus! Finally, someone told us to call her doctor. The doctor was well aware of her condition and convinced the EMS personnel to allow her to die. It was a mixture of sadness and relief when they finally stopped working on her. It was over. She was gone. They were all gone. Uncle Bob, Mom, Uncle Nicky, and Aunt Mary Jane. My mother's entire family had ceased to exist.

For the next several hours we waited in Mary Jane's apartment for the funeral director to come and remove her body. There she lay, dead in her bed, while we sat in her living room making funeral arrangements and struggling to make some sense of yet another loss. I couldn't help but look at her lying there, as if she would wake up any minute and make us a pot of her terrible coffee.

Journal Entry — Thursday, September 13, 1990
Talk about a nightmare! Aunt Mary Jane died Monday night while I was getting ready to go to her apartment. Thank God, Linda was with her when she took her last breath. The wake was yesterday and the funeral today. So many people from her co-op showed up and it really helped a lot. It has been an exhausting two days and I am very sad and somewhat numb. It seems so long ago that it all began. The mourning is just beginning. I will miss her so terribly. Sleep well, Motz.

My aunt's passing came seven years after my mother's, and in some ways it was much harder for me to accept. I was older now, married with a child and, unbeknownst to me at the time, another on the way. She was the last of the four Fraine siblings to die of cancer. In a span of just eight years, I had lost my mother and all my aunts and uncles. Now all of my mom's family was gone, and I was **angry**! We were all angry. All 12 of the Fraine cousins had lost a parent to cancer. It was beginning to look like more than just an unfortunate coincidence.

Sitting on that school bus after Aunt Mary Jane's funeral, I was reminded of the happier times. The Holy Communions, Confirmations and graduations we celebrated together. The weddings and new babies and Thanksgivings and Christmases. None of these joyous occasions would be the same without our parents around. I would miss the Bingo we played on holidays, the Sunday evening coffee and cake, and the banter of my mom and her sister and brothers as they shared the joys and sorrows of their lives.

Singing "Ninety-nine Bottles of Beer on the Wall" while riding through the cemetery was just the catharsis we all needed. It seemed like a fitting end to nearly a decade of pain and sorrow. But like the bottles on the wall, it wouldn't be long before another one would fall.

Part II

My Generation – The Wisdom of Vigilance

My Generation

Throughout the years of sickness and death our lives continued to move forward, though sometimes with sadness. There were still many happy occasions that we shared as a family. Laura married Jimmy in 1980, before we lost my mom and her siblings. She was the only sister to be that fortunate, but their first child wasn't born until after Mom was gone. Laura and Jimmy have three sons — Michael, Stephen and Andrew.

Linda and Al's wedding took place exactly three months after Mom's death, forcing Linda to reprint her wedding invitations to omit Mom's name. It was awful that such a happy occasion was marred by such grief, but in the end, their wedding proved to be a much-needed joyous event.

Journal Entry — Friday, May 13, 1983

Well, it's finally here. Linda's wedding is tomorrow and I'm feeling so many different things. Dad's really nervous and emotional and he's driving us all nuts. I hope we all have a good time tomorrow and not worry about everything or miss Mom too much. I'm excited, emotional and confused!

Linda and Al also have three sons — Albert, Christopher and Nicky. Three months after Linda's nuptials Jay and I became engaged, soon to leave just Carol and Dad in the somber house that was once an active, energetic home. In the midst of my elation over my impending marriage, I found it hard to shake the guilt over leaving Carol alone to pick up the pieces. Unselfishly, she was very supportive of us and graciously made it as easy as possible.

Journal Entry — August 13, 1983

What an incredible 36 hours just passed. Jay and I got engaged last night. He took me by hansom cab to Tavern on the Green and gave me the ring at dinner. Then we came home and told everyone. I'm thinking about Mom so much tonight and about how she would have reacted if she were alive.

I've grown up so much even since February, when she died. I'm not at all the same person, and my life has drastically changed. It's really so sad at times. I just don't know how Carol is going to live with Dad alone. I'd be so depressed if I were her. I feel like crying tonight just for the family we once were. How I wish I could go back and do it better. I wish I would have been closer to Mom instead of being afraid to talk to her. She was a wonderful, strong woman, and I hope I can carry her in my heart forever.

We were married the next year and Carol and Dad proceeded to live together with little conflict once they fell into a routine of sorts.

Journal Entry — November 26, 1984

Carol is doing much better than I ever expected. I can't believe how happy I am about that. When we got home from the honeymoon she had left champagne and wine and cheese in the apartment. Dad had us all over for dinner the first weekend we were home and I was walking on thin ice when I talked to Carol. I was really nervous that I would say something to offend her. Now it feels pretty normal again. I really want Carol to be happy.

Matthew was born to Jay and me in 1989, and one month after Aunt Mary Jane's death I discovered I was pregnant with our second son, Brian.

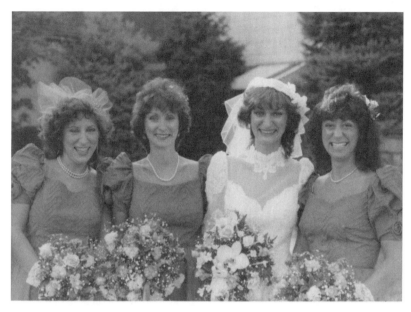

Celebrating Happy Times. My wedding day, September 1984. Left to right: Carol, Laura, Me, Linda.

Carol met George shortly after I was married. Their romance progressed quickly and they were married in 1987. Carol and George have two daughters. Carissa and Alana provide the much-needed feminine counterpoint to all the male cousins!

So the next generation begins. The four Tropea girls gave birth to eight sons and two daughters, and my mother never got to meet any of them. Only after all our children were born did we realize that we carried a deadly gene.

A Threat Becomes Reality

While still mourning our loved ones, Linda happened across an article about the Strang Cancer Prevention Center in New York City. Strang deals primarily with families at high risk for breast cancer. Since we could no longer deny the fact that we were high-risk, my sisters and I became part of the center's early surveillance program. At Strang's suggestion, we all began getting our yearly mammograms and breast exams while still well below the recommended age for the general population. In addition to being taught how to properly examine our own breasts, we were given a small plastic "test" breast with a lump inside. This "test" breast would enable us to differentiate between the feel of a tumor and the regular abnormalities of a healthy breast. In my case, it may have saved my life.

With the sadness and horror of the 1980s behind us, we all settled into life again. I was doing everything in my power to take care of my health. I tried to eat right and exercise. I didn't smoke and was only a social drinker. I had my yearly checkups and mammograms and did my breast self-exam every month. Things were going to be okay. Maybe there was something in my mom's drinking water growing up. Or perhaps my grandmother was exposed to something while she was pregnant, causing cancer in her children. I came up with a million reasons to dispel my own fears. After all, the cancer was in their generation, not mine.

We would have three years of false security before cancer struck again. This time it was in our generation!

Patty

My cousin Patty was diagnosed in 1993. Patty is Uncle Bob's daughter. At 40, she was diagnosed years younger than the others. We were all panic-stricken. I remember wondering, *NOW what? How can this be happening again? She has an adolescent daughter, for heaven's sake! How is poor Sarah going to be able to understand losing her mother? And from my own experiences with cancer, she WILL lose her. That's the way it works —isn't it? First you are diagnosed. Then they operate. Maybe they'll throw some chemotherapy and radiation in for good measure, but ultimately it will spread. Then you die.*

I had seen it before ... many times before. This was just too much to bear. I was terrified for Patty. Terrified for her husband, Jim. Terrified for Sarah. And yes, I'm not ashamed to admit, terrified for myself.

But then something happened that had never before happened in my family: Patty didn't die! She didn't die! She was the first one. They operated, as they did with the others. They did chemotherapy, as they did with the others. She lost all her hair, as did the others. But she didn't die! She got better. Her strength came back. Her hair grew back. Her life went on. She survived. She was a breast cancer survivor! There was hope. Thank God, there was hope!

New Discoveries

While one after another of my family was diagnosed with cancer, science was making new discoveries. In 1994 and 1995, researchers isolated two genes (called BRCA1 and BRCA2) that they believed might influence the development of breast cancer. Genes are present in the cells that make up our bodies and control everything from hair color to the enzymes that help us digest our food. Abnormalities in the genes are called *mutations*.

Individuals who carry mutations in the genes BRCA1 and BRCA2 are thought to be at an increased susceptibility for breast cancer, possibly as high as a 55–85 percent lifetime risk. The mutant genes also substantially increase the risk of ovarian cancer in women up to 40 percent, and elevate the risk of prostate cancer in men.

This was indeed a breakthrough discovery, but I wasn't sure how I would benefit from it. Most breast cancer is not caused by gene mutations, and most women who get breast cancer do not even have a family history of the disease. In fact, only 5–10 percent of breast cancer can be attributed to gene mutations. Nevertheless, genetic testing for the BRCA1 and BRCA2 mutations had now become available.

Testing for the genes should be performed only after genetic counseling, since there are many implications. It is suggested for those with a strong family history, such as families in which two or more close family members have been diagnosed with breast or ovarian cancer, in which breast cancer has been diagnosed before the age of 50, in which a male has been diagnosed with breast cancer, and families with Ashkenazi Jewish ancestry.

The test is performed by drawing a sample of blood and sending it to a laboratory, where it is analyzed. If the test is positive, the options are then discussed with the genetic counselor and the referring physician. Although the risk of developing breast cancer can be as high as 85 percent if a gene mutation is present, a positive test result does not mean that you will get breast cancer, nor does a negative result mean that you will not. Women with negative results can still develop breast cancer. Other genes not yet known, or not ordinarily tested for, can also account for familial disease.

The test itself is costly and not always covered by medical insurance. Many people who undergo genetic testing risk discrimination in insurance, employment and other areas. Because of these factors, genetic testing is confidential

So now I had another decision to make. Was genetic testing right for me? Back to the Strang Cancer Prevention Center we went. Four sisters, all terrified at the prospect of a positive test result, but equally frightened of remaining ignorant. It didn't seem as if there was a choice in the matter. We just had to find out more about this.

Our visit to Strang proved to be very informative. Genetic testing was still relatively new at that time. The counselor stressed the importance of thoroughly thinking it through before making any decisions. What would I do with the information once I had obtained it? Until now, close screening and early detection were the two most important factors in surviving breast cancer, and I already did those things. Why would I need to know more? That's when they laid the bombshell on us.

Strang informed us about new evidence indicating that prophylactic, or preventive, mastectomy (removal of both healthy breasts before the onset of cancer) for women at high risk can dramatically reduce the chances of developing the disease — by at least 90 percent!

But even with all this information available to me, I still kept coming back to the same question: Why? Why would I want to know if I have these mutant genes?

A negative test wouldn't guarantee that I won't get breast cancer in the future. And if I were to test positive, what would I do? My options were: increased screening, monthly self-exams, yearly mammograms and a basic diet and exercise regimen — all of which I already practiced. And the idea of removing perfectly healthy breasts as a precaution seemed like an incredibly drastic move. Aside from the obvious physical changes, there would be psychological aspects as well. I didn't think that the procedure would remove the nagging doubt that I might have taken the drastic step for naught. I was sure that with all the recent breakthroughs in medicine, a less invasive precaution would become available in the near future.

The four of us listened intently to the counselor and formed our own opinions. Linda felt rather strongly that she would like to proceed with genetic testing. Laura and Carol were undecided. I was vehemently against it. Genetic testing was not for me! We were all in agreement, however, that more research was needed and that none of us were ready to proceed with genetic testing at that time. So, once again, life proceeded normally . . . for a while.

My Diagnosis

In July of 1998 things were going very well in my life. Having just completed 3rd grade, Matthew was 9 years old. Brian, age 7, had just completed 1st grade. Both were "A" students. They were still young enough to love Jay and me unconditionally, yet old enough to be relatively self-sufficient.

Jay's job was going well, although he traveled more than either of us would have liked. As for me, after more years than I care to admit, I was anxiously awaiting my college diploma in the mail. We were thoroughly enjoying parenthood and had a full summer, complete with several vacations, ahead of us.

Then it happened.

During a self-exam, I felt a lump in my left breast. It felt different from any other lumps or bumps I had felt in my breasts before. I showed it to Jay immediately. I could see the blood drain from his face when he felt it. He knew as well as I did that this was something different. I pulled out my mini test breast and was devastated to discover that it felt exactly the same.

Without hesitation, I was off to my gynecologist. To my surprise and delight, my doctor was "not impressed" with the lump. But as luck would have it, she recently had begun sharing office space with a surgeon down the hall, so she sent him in to have a look. Well, the surgeon *was* impressed with the lump. He told me that since he and I could both feel it, and it shouldn't be there, we should probably do something about it. He told me that I had two options. I could wait six months to see if it went away, or I could have it biopsied immediately. He suggested I go home and discuss it with my husband. Well, there was not a doubt in my mind what I wanted to do. I told him that no discussion was necessary; I wanted it biopsied right away! Who knows what could happen in six months?

The biopsy was performed in the surgeon's office on July 7, 1998. It would be several days before I got the results. For some reason, I wasn't that nervous. In fact, it was my dad who encouraged me to keep calling the doctor before the weekend arrived. So, as I was heading home from the beach with my two little boys in the car, the doctor called on my cell phone with the diagnosis. Malignant. It was *malignant!*

A million thoughts ran through my head. I was frantic. *How could this be? I am only 38 years old. How will I explain it to my kids? They still need me — how can I leave them? Dying just isn't an option right now, I'm not done yet. Doesn't that stupid doctor know that? This is only supposed to happen to other people, not to me.* But it did happen to me. I had breast cancer. My luck had run out. I was about to enter the fight of my life.

I can barely remember the rest of the ride home. I do recall that I got off at the wrong exit and just started driving around aimlessly. At one point I picked up the cell phone and called Jay at work. "Can you come home?" was all I had to say. He knew immediately that the news was bad.

Once I arrived home, I called the doctor back. He told me about my options. I could either have a lumpectomy with radiation, or I could opt for a mastectomy. There would be bone scans, MRIs, mammograms, *blah, blah, blah.* My brain could barely comprehend all that he was telling me. I'd need to see a plastic surgeon and an oncologist, *blah, blah, blah.* How was I supposed to handle all this? I needed to talk to someone! I needed to see Jay! I needed to hug my kids! Dear God, please, I needed to have this all go away! An hour ago I was driving home from a nice day at the beach and now I'm a cancer patient. How could this be?

Eventually I calmed myself down enough to start calling my family. I began by calling Linda, whom I had just left at the beach. She gasped when she heard the news. I asked that she spread the word.

Next, I called my cousin Patty. It had been nearly six years since her diagnosis and she was still cancer-free. She was also the only person in

my family who actually had *survived* cancer. I needed to speak to someone who had been there and lived to tell about it. Patty's first words
were "I'm sorry. No one ever said *I'm sorry* to me when I was diagnosed,
and I want you to know that I am truly sorry that you have to face this."

Patty went on to give me some idea of what I could expect to hear
in regard to surgery and treatment. I questioned her on everything —
chemotherapy, mastectomy, lumpectomy, and every other term that was
being tossed around. She told me of her experience as best she could,
without frightening me further. It was comforting to know that she
had been through breast cancer and it was now just a distant memory
for her.

As the news began to spread, everyone started calling me. For some
reason I became frighteningly calm. I asked the same of my family, that
they remain calm and that they never show any shock or fear at anything that was to come. I knew with certainty that my life was forever
changed from that day forward.

It was a couple of hours before Jay was able to make his way from
his Manhattan office to our Long Island home in the Friday afternoon
traffic. By the time he got home, I had somehow managed to shower
and change. The kids were outside playing with friends. They knew
nothing of the curse that had just befallen their family. To outsiders, it
was business as usual in the Greene household.

Jay walked into the bedroom and we just held each other. My first
concern was for our kids. I couldn't imagine how we were all going to
get through this. As usual, Jay's mere presence made me stronger. He
told me that we were in this fight together and that we would win. I
often wonder what I would have done without him.

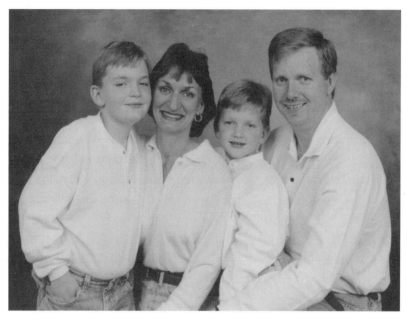

My "Hurry Up Before I Die" Picture. Taken shortly after my diagnosis in October 1998. Matthew, me, Brian and Jay.

Jay

I never really believed people who claimed that they married their best friend, but that's exactly what I did. In fact, I never thought that Jay would be anything but my best friend. I certainly never thought he would become my husband!

I was 8 years old when my family moved from the Bronx to Queens. Jay, who was also 8, lived with his family right next door. Our houses even shared a common driveway. We became part of the same crowd of kids in the neighborhood. I remember the seemingly endless summer days spent playing games like kickball and stickball in the street, and going in the neighbor's pool or to the beach. Jay was always part of it. He and I became friends despite his shy and sometimes awkward demeanor with girls.

Throughout high school I had a steady boyfriend, but Jay was still part of my life. We would "call for" one another when either of us was free. We'd talk about everything — parents, school, relationships, and our dreams for the future. No subject was taboo. He always opened up with me and we continued to grow closer. I was even his date for his high school senior prom. He was my buddy, my confidant, my best friend. He would *never* be my boyfriend. Jay was the person in whom I'd *confide* about my boyfriend. Although he wanted to pursue taking our relationship to the next level, we remained platonic friends.

After high school I went on to my first full-time job. I was commuting to Manhattan every day and meeting new people from all walks of life. I was making money, traveling, and even dating an "older man." Jay was attending college and also dating someone new. Our friendship began to wane. I mistakenly assumed that he was still the shy, quiet boy I knew from next door, while I fancied myself a "working woman." There was no way he would catch up with me now!

Some years went by and it was becoming obvious to me that I was in an unhealthy relationship with my boyfriend. My friends were graduating from college and I was beginning to regret never having gone. Jay was struggling in his relationship as well. He had graduated from college and had moved into an apartment of his own. One day we ran into one another and, realizing that we were both free that night, decided to go out for a drink. We talked all night, commiserating about our respective relationships and catching up on what was going on in our lives. After that night, I began to look at Jay differently; maybe he *could* be more than just a friend.

It was a slow process, but I finally opened my eyes in time to realize that Jay was much more than just the "kid" next door. While I was waiting for *him* to grow up, it turned out that I was the one who needed to mature! He encouraged me to go back to school and stood by my side during my mother's illness and ultimate death, all the while asking nothing in return. Jay taught me what it means to truly love someone. He became, and still is, the love of my life, the person without whom I never could have gotten through my cancer experience. He gives me love, guidance, support, optimism and, most of all, humor. Yes, I married my best friend.

Absorbing the Shock

In the first days and weeks following my diagnosis, Jay and I attempted to keep our lives as normal as possible. We accepted his brother's invitation to a barbecue the very first weekend. We had hoped to find some comfort in being with family and friends, but when I saw the fear and helplessness in everyone's eyes upon our arrival, I immediately knew we had made a mistake. After trying in vain to make idle conversation, I finally excused myself and went upstairs to a bedroom to lie down. My head was pounding and I could no longer pretend that things were going to be okay.

Through the open window I could hear our kids laughing and playing with their cousins, without a care in the world. *Innocent kids*, I thought. *They have no idea that their mother is dying.* In the background I could also hear Jay's voice as he attempted to find some normalcy in this whole ordeal. *And Jay. . . he's going to be known as the young widower left to raise his two small sons alone!*

I was convinced that I would never again know happiness. Never have another carefree day in my life or be able to laugh with Jay and the kids the way we so often did. I was crippled with sadness — mourning my own inevitable death. I stayed in the bedroom wallowing in self-pity for more than an hour.

I tried to sleep away reality, but there was too much noise outside. So many people talking and laughing. So many people having fun. *How can they be having fun while I'm up here dying?* Maybe I wasn't actually *dying*, but

I was certainly *going* to die. Wasn't I? I was so angry at the cancer. It had taken so many innocent lives. So many of those I loved had been struck down by this horrible beast.

As I lay there feeling sorry for myself, the memory of those who had battled the disease before me came into my mind. I started to think about Angela and how bravely she had faced her cancer so many years earlier.

Angela Volpe and I went to the same grade school, but our friendship really blossomed when we shared the same home room in high school. Born just one day apart, she and I always celebrated our birthdays together. Angela started battling Hodgkin's disease at the tender age of 16. When we traveled together to Hawaii after our 18th birthdays, she had already been rendered sterile by her chemotherapy regimen and was wearing a wig to cover her bald head. Still, she would don wild bandanas when we went to the beach, and joke about scaring the housekeepers with her wig — affectionately nicknamed *Wilma* — which she hung on the television antenna in our hotel room. Even after the airline lost her luggage, Angela was determined to make the most of our long-awaited vacation. Hoisting up my size 9 shorts onto her petite size 3 frame, she went about enjoying our Hawaiian holiday.

I remember the time that I was complaining incessantly to her about some trivial matter that seemed catastrophic to my 18-year-old mind. Upon realizing that she had significantly more important things to worry about, I shamefully apologized for my lack of consideration. She turned to me and said, "Don't ever apologize because you think my problems are bigger than yours. Yours may be smaller, but they are still problems to you, and therefore equally important." Angela died a little more than a year later, but the memory of her courage and determination has stayed with me.

Then, of course, there was my mother and her sister and brothers, fighting so hard to live. My mother never gave up, she *never* let the cancer defeat her. She dealt with it daily and went on with her life. It may have *killed* her, but it never *defeated* her. If nothing else, I had to honor the memory of my family and friends who had fought their cancer battles so fearlessly. I owed it to my children and my husband.

I had two choices. I could lie there defeated, wasting my life waiting for the cancer to kill me. Or I could get up, stop feeling sorry for myself, and get ready for the fight of my life! Life wasn't going to stop because I had cancer.

I pulled myself together and went back outside.

Forging the Battle

Together Jay and I entered a new stage in our lives where our days became a blur of tests and appointments. In the beginning I couldn't even say the words aloud. *Breast cancer. . . breast cancer. . .* no I couldn't have breast cancer! I wouldn't let Jay say it either. I asked him to refer to it as a malignant tumor — not breast cancer! It was as if by not saying the words, the cancer wasn't a reality. The same was true for writing it down. I'll never forget filling out the first form. You know those boxes — have you ever had . . . *Heart disease?* No. *Asthma?* No. *High blood pressure?* No. *Seizures?* No. *Cancer?* **Cancer?** **Cancer?** Okay, okay . . . yes . . . I have *cancer!* Are you happy now? It took a while to sink in, but, like it or not, I had cancer.

There was so much to do and remember. No matter how hard we tried, it was starting to overwhelm us. Breast surgeons, oncologists and plastic surgeons. Telephone numbers and appointments to remember, insurance questions to have answered, and terms and procedures to understand. On top of the emotional strain of my being newly diagnosed with breast cancer, we were deluged with new information to explore and decipher.

In a frenzied attempt to remain in control, Jay set out to purchase a notebook to help organize all the data we were acquiring. It was covered in green fabric with a Velcro closure. The front cover had a zipper pocket to store business cards, and the lined pages inside were divided into sections. I made a separate section for *breast surgeons, oncologists,* insurance, and plastic surgeons. Prior to an appointment I would list all my questions and concerns, so I could jot down the answers when I spoke to the doctor. At home I would reread everything and rewrite it using a layperson's terms. If I succeeded in deciphering my notes, I knew that I had a complete understanding. Doing this helped us to make sense of everything we were being told, and seeing it written in my own hand simplified it and took away some of the anxiety. As long as I had my little green "security blanket" with me, everything seemed to make sense.

With notebook in hand we were off to see our first breast surgeon. She was a tall, no-nonsense, take-charge woman, and I liked her right away. Jay was seated in the room with me as she did a thorough examination of my breasts. I could see him squirming in his seat, not knowing where to look. When she left the room for a moment, he turned to me and said, "Gee, this was always my fantasy, but under these circumstances, it didn't quite live up to my expectations!" We both burst out laughing. Jay could always make me laugh, and I realized then that with him by my side, we would get through this.

After examining me and reading through my lab reports, the surgeon suggested a lumpectomy (the removal of the tumor and surrounding tissue), with radiation. I was skeptical at first, uncertain that a lumpectomy was the way to go. *Why leave any breast tissue? Wouldn't it be better to remove the whole breast?* While I certainly didn't desire a larger surgery, a part of me felt like screaming, "Just chop the damn thing off!" Since puberty, my breasts had caused me nothing but heartache; it was if they had a mind of their own. They had taunted me throughout my adolescence and now they were threatening to kill me!

You Win the Kewpie Doll

At around age 9 or 10, my girlfriends and I couldn't wait to get our first bras. It was the symbol that we were becoming *women*. I can remember going into the store and looking longingly at the bra section. *Who would be the first one to get a bra? Would it be one of those flat "training bras" or a real one, with cups?* We fantasized about the day it would finally happen.

Getting our first bras was an exciting event. Mine was a training bra — size 28AA. Basically, that means that you don't need a bra at all, but if you *must* wear one, size 28AA is the smallest one you can buy. As we matured into our teens, our girlish discussions turned away from training bras and onto more serious topics — like boys and dating. Wearing a bra was just something young women did; it certainly wasn't anything to talk about. So it came as a surprise to me when our discussions turned back to the size of our bras — the size of my bra in particular.

While I was busy growing up and dealing with my typical teenage insecurities, I began to develop much faster, and quite a bit larger, than most of my girlfriends. If you were to ask anyone who knew me in my teens to give you one defining feature about me, chances are they would say my breasts.

Much to my dismay, I became known as the girl with the "big tits." While the rest of my figure was slender, by the time I was 16 I was wearing a size DD bra! I **hated** it! Most of my girlfriends were jealous and most of the guys were delighted. No one ever considered my feelings as they teased me or made lewd comments. I was tormented so much at a party once that I hauled off and slapped a guy across the face.

I could never find anything to fit me properly. While the other girls were wearing the popular styles of the '70s, like tube tops and halters, I was stuck wearing T-shirts. They would buy sexy little stretch bras with matching lace panties, while I was forced to shop in the "old lady" section of the lingerie department. The bras that fit me properly were displayed in boxes near the girdles and were fraught with underwire, thick straps and elastic claiming to "lift and separate." And there was not a matching lace panty to be found!

Buying swimwear was always a project. My mother and I would scour the racks to find a bathing suit suitable for a large-breasted girl, yet youthful enough to be stylish and age-appropriate. With all the time I spent on the beach in the summer, it was difficult to remain indistinguishable among the other girls. When a total stranger approached me and announced, loud enough for his buddies to hear, "Congratulations, you win the kewpie doll for having the biggest tits on the beach," I wanted to bury myself in the sand and disappear! So my initial instinct to tell the doctor to take off my breast came as no surprise to me.

My painful teenage insecurities were replaced with the promise of a less extensive surgery once I started meeting with doctors. After three separate breast surgeons concurred that a lumpectomy was the best course of treatment in my case, I became secure in my decision. Numerous studies had shown that for early stage breast cancer, a lumpectomy with radiation was equivalent to mastectomy in terms of survival.

Journal Entry — Monday, July 20, 1998

I'm amazed that it's taken me this long to sit down and write about this horror story. Two weeks ago I found a lump in my breast. Last Friday I was told it was malignant. I've been to two doctors so far and both have suggested a lumpectomy with radiation. Tomorrow I am going to Sloan Kettering to see another one. I am a nervous wreck right now because I am totally confused. If he has a different opinion, I think I'll just scream!

Journal Entry — Tuesday, July 21, 1998

Things are going to be OK. I went to Sloan Kettering today and the surgeon agreed with everything the other two doctors said. It was the peace of mind I needed to help me make this decision. I feel fairly confident that things are going to be fine.

In addition to the lumpectomy, the doctors suggested a procedure called *sentinel node biopsy*. They explained that the lymph nodes under the armpit are an integral part of a breast cancer diagnosis. In the past, surgeons removed all or most of the lymph nodes in a procedure called *axillary node dissection*, in order to test them for cancer. The presence of cancer cells in the lymph nodes and the number of lymph nodes that contain cancer determine, along with the size of the lump, the stage of the cancer. The stage then determines the best course of treatment. The problem with axillary node dissection is that it potentially has significant long-lasting side effects, the worst of which is *lymphedema*.

Lymphedema is a chronic swelling of the arm that often requires physical therapy to keep under control. Stiffness of the shoulder and numbness on the back of the upper arm are other problems. These side effects do not occur in the majority of patients. If they do occur, they can be mild, intermediate or even severe. My mom and my aunt had axillary node dissections when they were diagnosed, and both suffered from painful swelling and limited movement of their arms. Thus, the sentinel node biopsy was certainly something to consider. Since many people with early stage breast cancer have negative lymph nodes, this procedure avoids removal of many normal nodes in those cases and could eliminate or at least lessen those problems for me.

In this procedure, prior to surgery two different tracer materials are injected into the breast near the site of the tumor or underneath the nipple area. One material is radioactive (a very low, non-dangerous dose), and the second is a blue dye. The sentinel node is located by using a special probe in the operating room to detect radioactivity, or by seeing which node turns blue. Sometimes one node is both radioactive and blue; at other times two or three nodes pick up either one or both of the tracers. Each of these nodes must then be removed and examined to determine if the cancer has spread. The assumption is that cancer cells follow the same pathway as the tracer materials.

If the sentinel nodes are free of cancer, the rest of the lymph nodes are assumed to be unaffected as well, thus eliminating the need for their removal. However, if there is cancer in the sentinel nodes it is important to know how many nodes are affected, and the standard axillary dissection is then performed.

After weeks of appointments and hours of research and deliberation, Jay and I had settled on the surgery best for me. I was scheduled for a lumpectomy with sentinel node biopsy on August 3, 1998. Though confident about the type of surgery, we were still dealing with lingering trepidation over what might be uncovered once they removed more breast tissue. There were still so many unknowns. *What if there's cancer in the nodes? What if the tumor is larger than they thought? What if? What if? What if?* There were a million *what ifs.* While we wallowed in our plight, a telephone call would bring us news so unspeakable it would snap us back to the present and help us realize there were problems far greater than ours.

A car accident had taken the life of our friend's 14-year-old daughter. Poor Sarah never had a chance. On the way to a concert with a friend, her young life was snuffed out by a speeding car. There was no drinking. There were no drugs. There was no irresponsible behavior on her part. The victim of a careless driver, she was guilty only of being in the wrong place at the wrong time. Now this was a tragedy! To say goodbye to your child one minute and the next minute see a grim-faced police officer at your door with his hat in his hand was inconceivable to me.

Right then and there I decided that my own fate was out of my hands. I would do whatever I had to do to regain my health, but worrying would get me nowhere. The grave fate of a young girl would give me strength. Sarah turned out to be my angel.

With young Sarah's smiling face and news of the terrible accident splashed across the headlines the next morning, my heart was heavy as I entered the hospital for my lumpectomy. The surgery went smoothly and without complications, and I was home the same night. At only °cm. (about ˜ inch), my tumor was very small. Thankfully, the preliminary pathology report showed that the lymph nodes were benign, likely signifying the cancer had not spread, although a final pathology report was expected in a week or so. But along with this so-called good news was some not-so-good news.

The examination of the lumpectomy tissue uncovered something called *ductal carcinoma in situ* (DCIS). DCIS refers to cancer cells that are still within the ducts of the breast. All of it must be removed to provide the best chance for cure. Sometimes this can be accomplished by a second lumpectomy, but often the best option is removal of the entire breast by mastectomy. My doctor felt strongly that my case warranted a total mastectomy. *Aaaarrgghhh! Wasn't that my initial instinct?* I wrestled with the impulse to second-guess our decision for the lumpectomy, although the truth was simply that I was disturbed to be prolonging the whole process and adding another surgery to the mix as well. I wanted to be done with it. This "summer of surgery" was droning on, and it was becoming increasingly more difficult to keep a stiff upper lip. And, astonishing as it may sound, I wasn't the only one in my family who was facing the terror of cancer.

During that same time period, Linda was preparing to undergo surgery on what appeared to be a very large mass on her ovary, and Laura was scheduled for a biopsy on two spots discovered on her breast. What are the chances of three sisters having cancer scares at the same time? If this hadn't been happening in my own family, I wouldn't have believed it.

Journal Entry — Thursday, August 6, 1998

Had my surgery on Monday and everything went well, but I am still waiting for the final pathology report that will determine if the cancer has spread or not. Carol stayed over Sunday and Monday and really helped me out a lot. People have been great. I got tons of flowers and cards. It really makes me feel great.

Linda has a "mass" on either her ovary or uterus which they just discovered today. She's scheduled for an MRI next Friday. It's almost too much to be true. Laura goes in for a biopsy on two spots on her breast tomorrow. Isn't this almost laughable?

Before scheduling the mastectomy, Jay and I felt strongly that we should still go on our annual vacation to Ocean City, Maryland. It was something we really wanted to do for ourselves as well as for the kids. It had been a hell of a summer so far, and we all really needed some normalcy in our lives. After all, we weren't the only ones feeling the magnitude of the cancer. Our vacation buddies, the "Friday Night Pizza Group," had been down this road as well.

"Friday Night Pizza Group" was a silly little name that evolved after years of getting together with friends every Friday night for pizza. When the kids were little and it was difficult to plan an evening out, it became the perfect way to see one another. The kids played together while we adults sat down over a glass of wine and pizza to catch up and have a few laughs. Everyone would bring something, maybe wine, beer or dessert, as we rotated among our houses each week.

When it began, the group consisted of Richie and Charlotte, Stew and Teresa, Rosie and Rob, Sally and Steve, and Jay and me, along with all our kids. We had been through a lot together — births, a miscarriage, childhood diseases and ailing parents. We also had faced the death of one of us.

Stew was diagnosed with liver and pancreatic cancer two years earlier, in July 1996. By the time his cancer was discovered, it had already progressed to a deadly stage. Stew never had a chance. Just six weeks later he lost his battle, leaving behind his wife, Teresa, and three beautiful young daughters.

Watching the strength Stew displayed as he faced his impending death was extraordinary. At just 38 years old, he still had so much ahead of him. He longed to grow old with Teresa and watch his daughters become women, but the doctors were unable to give him any hope of survival. Somehow Stew still faced his death with grace, poise and, in his words, "quiet acceptance." Though I couldn't have known it at the time, I would draw on Stew's strength and dignity many times as I was going through my own cancer experience. So along with young Sarah, Angela, and the family I had already lost to cancer, Stew was another angel looking down upon me.

This would be the second summer that Teresa was strong enough to make the Ocean City vacation without Stew. The previous year had been melancholy, to say the least. This year would be marred by my cancer diagnosis, but that was all the more reason we felt we should go.

If Teresa was strong enough to tough it out, I would be too. I was lucky enough to have a good chance of survival and we'd be damned if we were going to let this cancer put a damper on our family vacation! So, armed with my green book, a cell phone and a beeper, we were off to the shore.

The familiar sounds and smells of the beach comforted me and lulled me into a safe place, if only for a while. For the most part, we were able to take some time out from the worries and stress that awaited us; however, we were still in constant contact back home. Linda was undergoing her biopsy, and I was awaiting the final pathology report that would tell me whether or not my cancer had spread to my lymph nodes.

We were on the beach when Jay's beeper sounded, signaling the long-awaited call from my breast surgeon's office with the final results. I motioned for Jay to get out of the water and we headed back up to our room in silence, to make the dreaded phone call. The lymph nodes were benign. They were *benign!* The final pathology results showed that there were no micro-metastases — meaning that under more extensive pathological examination, the nodes still showed no signs of cancer! We rushed down the hall to Teresa's room to tell her the good news. She jumped up and down with us as we all hugged and kissed in celebration. Then Jay and I ran down to the beach to tell the rest of our friends as Teresa watched from her balcony, yelling and waving frantically. It was a celebration of hope and survival that I will never forget.

Journal Entry — Monday, August 17, 1998

Sitting in our living room in Ocean City, and having a really nice time. It almost feels like I don't have any problems, but, boy, is that ever a joke! Linda is going in for her surgery today. I'll call Daddy later. I pray that it's benign. I just don't know what she's going to do if it's malignant.

Both Linda and Laura came out of their respective biopsies fine. Laura's was just another terrifying scare, of which she'd had many. And although Linda ended up having a complete hysterectomy, thankfully her tumor was benign. I don't think that our family would have been able to withstand anything else.

Once we returned from vacation, the frenetic pace resumed. The mastectomy was scheduled for September 1st and I was now considering removing my healthy breast along with my cancerous breast. I was going to have reconstructive surgery anyway, and the plastic surgeon mentioned that it would be easier to make both breasts "match" if they were removed simultaneously. I also couldn't stop worrying about the possibility that I had DCIS in the other breast.

My breast surgeon felt that, in the absence of genetic testing revealing a mutation, she would recommend removing both breasts if "it's the only way you can sleep at night." She felt that with a single mastectomy we could monitor the remaining breast with mammograms, sonograms and MRIs, in the hope of discovering any abnormalities at an early stage. It was all just too huge a decision to make at that point. I was terrified of the single mastectomy, and doubling it was just inconceivable. I settled on having the single mastectomy.

September 1st arrived and my mastectomy went as planned. When I awoke I was wearing a surgical bra that covered gauze and dressing underneath. This surgical bra looked much like a sports bra, with a Velcro closure in front.

I had chosen implant reconstruction, and my plastic surgeon had started the procedure during my mastectomy, but I would need two more surgeries to complete the process. During the mastectomy a temporary implant, called a "tissue expander," was put into place where my breast once was. In the coming weeks, saline would be injected into the expander by a needle inserted though the skin and into a valve in the expander. This would enable my skin to be stretched gradually. Several months later the tissue expander would be removed and the final implant would be inserted. Another procedure would add a nipple and areola.

The morning after my surgery, the plastic surgeon arrived to check on the surgical site. I had been focusing so much on removing the cancer, I hadn't begun to address the emotional impact of losing my breast. So when he ripped open the Velcro and removed the gauze, I was completely unprepared for what I saw!

My breast had been replaced with what is referred to as a "mound," formed by the tissue expander placed under my chest muscle. Since the expander was only partially filled, it created a very small semblance of a breast. The incision atop the mound was covered with white surgical tape called Steri-Strip skin closures. The Steri-Strip closures ran horizontally across the center of my new "breast," protecting the stitches and, thankfully, disguising the harsh reality that I no longer had a nipple.

It was a devastating blow to see the disfigurement the surgery had caused, but I remained hopeful that when the reconstruction process was completed I would feel whole again. More importantly, my cancerous left breast had become my enemy and we now had successfully annihilated my evil adversary!

I was released from the hospital just 24 hours after the surgery, and Jay took time off from work to care for me. Fortunately, I was in good health in every other respect, so my recovery went smoothly, although not without some pain.

I was sent home with a tube dangling from under my arm on the side where the breast was removed. On the end of the tube was an egg-shaped plastic bulb that collected the blood and fluids that would drain from the area for nearly a week. Every few hours I would have to record the amount of fluid collected and then empty the plastic bulb. This "drain" under my arm would pull and pinch and caused much discomfort. Additionally, I wasn't able to raise my arm above my head or pick up anything heavy.

The pain in the breast area was bearable and for the most part kept under control by painkillers. However, when I prematurely tried to wash and dry my hair, I paid for it with excruciating pain for the next several hours.

We had a tremendous outpouring of support from family and friends. People came out of the woodwork to help us out. Neighbors brought us food and ran errands for us. Since the kids spent a few days in New Jersey with my sister Carol, I was able to take it easy and put all my energy into recuperating. In fact, just five days later, Jay and I were walking on the boardwalk at the beach with our kids. It was beginning to look as if things were getting back to normal. But normal was going to take on a whole new meaning. Now I had to meet with an oncologist to determine whether or not chemotherapy was in order.

Chemotherapy

The first oncologist I visited did not think chemotherapy would be in my best interest. He felt that chemo would probably increase my already 90 percent survival rate by about 1 percent. This was not a significant increase in his mind, and he felt that the benefits did not outweigh the risks. While I was thrilled with this news, off I went to another oncologist for a second opinion. I needed confirmation that I was doing the right thing.

On October 15, 1998, my 39th birthday, I went for my second opinion. I thought that it was an open-and-shut case. I was just going to walk into the office and be told that there was no need for chemo. No such luck. This second doctor was much more conservative and felt that chemo would definitely benefit me. *Now what do I do?* This opened up a whole new cause for concern. There was so much to consider.

Journal Entry — Thursday, October 15, 1998
I'm 39 today. I wonder how many more birthdays I am going to have? I've been running around so much lately to sort of "run away" from the cancer. Maybe if I keep moving, it won't catch me. I'm going to the oncologist tonight to discuss everything at length.

Because chemotherapy drugs are strong enough to kill stray cancer cells, they also kill some healthy cells. There was a good chance I would go into premature menopause and even lose all my hair. Chemo can cause nausea, vomiting and lethargy, and one pamphlet mentioned that in very rare cases it can even cause leukemia! Was I trading one disease for another? This was the toughest decision I had to make regarding the cancer thus far! It frightened me more than the two surgeries I'd already had and the two I knew were in my future. I very rarely even took a Tylenol for a headache and now I had to decide whether or not to put toxic drugs directly into my veins!

Days turned into weeks as we frantically tried to meet with a third oncologist to help us make a decision. When we finally sat down with her, she began spewing statistics in recent studies comparing treatment with and without chemo. It was all just too much to comprehend. Finally I asked her directly, "With your knowledge of cancer, if it were you, would you have chemo?" She thought about it for a minute and then replied, "Yes, I would." That was all I needed to hear to make my decision crystal clear. I would have the chemo.

There are as many different types of chemotherapy as there are types of cancer. The next thing we had to decide was which type of chemo would be right for me. Since my tumor was only ° cm. and I had no lymph node involvement, the doctors considered this preventive chemotherapy. I was thrilled to discover that the type of drugs prescribed were relatively mild.

Chemotherapy for breast cancer is most often a combination of drugs given intravenously to reduce the chance that the cancer will return. In my case, the protocol called for eight treatments of chemo, given intravenously every three weeks. It would take a total of six months to complete.

The type of chemo I was given was called CMF — cyclophosphamide (Cytoxan), methotrexate, and 5-fluorouracil (5 FU). The combination of these three drugs, the oncologist felt, would give me the best chance at a longer survival without having as toxic an effect as some other drugs. There were still many possible side effects, the most severe being early menopause, but I was ready to take on this new challenge. I wanted to be sure I did everything in my power to rid my body of this horrendous disease. I had come this far, so what was another six months?

Journal Entry — Tuesday, November 3, 1998

Saw another oncologist. She said I don't "need" the chemo either, but I know in my heart I should. I will begin as soon as I'm fully recovered from the reconstruction, which I am getting on the 19th. I feel very comfortable with this decision now that I've finally made it. They say I have a 40 percent chance of some thinning of my hair. I got my hair cut short today, my "chemo cut." It looks OK and should help a bit if my hair thins.

Before starting the chemo, I had the second stage of the reconstructive surgery. In November my plastic surgeon performed what is called the "implant exchange" — the removal of the tissue expander and insertion of the saline implant. I was thrilled to have this done and to be through with my weekly "fill-ups," but I still had to have the third and final surgery once I was through with the chemo.

Journal Entry — Tuesday, November 12, 1998

Spent the whole morning at the hospital for pre-op testing. I'm very, very nervous about this operation. It shouldn't be nearly as bad as the mastectomy (which wasn't even bad), but I am still nervous. Guess I just don't have much fight left in me.

The implant-exchange surgery was performed on November 19th. The surgery was really no big deal and I was thrilled to be done with it. Now I was almost whole again. At least I didn't have to keep traveling to the plastic surgeon's office every week.

Journal Entry — Tuesday, November 24, 1998

Well, I had the reconstructive surgery on the 19th. I calmed down a bit beforehand, finally. It was actually no big deal. The anesthesia was a terrible experience, though. My mouth was so dry that I choked on whatever I tried to eat the first 24 hours afterward. By Friday night I was finally OK. The breast pain isn't too bad. When I finally unveiled myself Friday afternoon it looked pretty good.

I've been weepy all day. I'm nervous about the chemo and starting to really feel like a cancer patient. On the other hand I am so thankful for my beautiful family and friends, and so excited about a lot of fun things we have coming up. I want to keep really busy because when I slow down it all seems to fall on top of me.

I started my chemo on December 10, 1998, six months after my diagnosis. I scheduled my appointments on Thursdays while the kids were in school. Jay was able to take me to all but one of my treatments.

Initially, chemotherapy was a terrifying experience. I was put in the "chemo room" with all the other cancer patients — many of them bald and looking tired, pale and afraid. It was a horrible place, with everyone hooked up to an IV. *I don't belong here! These people are sick, I'm not one of them!* But as time went on I came to realize that I, too, was a cancer patient, that I was very much like the rest of the people there. We were all fighting for our lives. Although sometimes a discouraged or defeated person sat in that room, for the most part we all realized that this was actually a good thing. It was a frightening and humbling experience, but in the end the chemotherapy was going to lengthen and enhance our lives. I chose to look at it as a positive thing.

Each treatment took about two to three hours. The nurses were very caring and informative, telling me what each drug was and what I could expect to feel as each one was put into my IV. Jay sat with me at each treatment. Sometimes we would watch TV or just talk. Sometimes I would doze off. After each treatment we would go out to lunch. It was as if we were on a date. He would take the whole day off and we would spend it together. Never mind the reason — we were together and that was all that mattered. Shortly after we returned home, the kids would come home from school. They always knew when it was my "chemo day," but we kept the details to ourselves.

Because I was given a low dose of chemo, I tolerated it remarkably well. Once or twice I had some mouth sores, but that was the extent of it. I never felt tired or nauseated and I didn't lose my hair. As far as chemotherapy goes, I realize that I was one of the very lucky ones. Still, each treatment was another reminder that I was "sick" and I just longed to put it all behind me and return to my normal life. In the weeks in between, I would give myself shots of a drug called Neupogen to ensure that my blood counts were high enough to withstand the next treatment. It was a cruel reminder that I was still a cancer *patient*. Oh, how I longed to be a cancer *survivor*.

Jay and I approached each session as another milestone accomplished, and before we knew it I was done! My last treatment was in May 1999. I would have my final reconstructive surgery in June, and then I would be done and could put this all behind me... right? Wrong. Oh, I was so very wrong.

Journal Entry — Wednesday, May 12, 1999

I had my last chemo on May 6th. I am so very glad that it's over. I am scheduled for the last surgery on June 11th. I really can't wait! While I am thrilled that things are coming to an end, I am also a bit nervous. I feel that if I let my guard down it's going to creep up on me again.

Once the chemotherapy was completed, I had another decision to make. My oncologist informed me about a drug called tamoxifen. Tamoxifen is a medication in pill form that interferes with the activity of estrogen. Estrogen can aid in the growth of estrogen receptor– positive tumors. When used as an adjuvant therapy, tamoxifen helps prevent the return of the original breast cancer and also helps prevent the development of new cancers in the other breast. (Adjuvant therapies are given to prevent cancer recurrence, without knowing whether there are actually any cancer cells present.)

My doctor felt that I was a good candidate for this drug since my tumor was estrogen receptor–positive, meaning that my tumor's growth might be stimulated by estrogen. Tamoxifen acts *against* the effects of estrogen in breast tissue, while it acts *like* estrogen in other tissues. This means that women who take tamoxifen may derive many of the beneficial effects of estrogen replacement therapy, such as lower blood cholesterol and slower bone loss (osteoporosis).

Unfortunately, there are also many adverse reactions associated with tamoxifen. In general, the side effects are similar to some of the symptoms of menopause. The most common are hot flashes and vaginal discharge. Some women also experience irregular menstrual periods, headaches, fatigue, nausea, vaginal dryness and skin rashes. More importantly, the drug increases the risk of two types of cancer that can develop in the uterus: endometrial cancer, which arises in the lining of the uterus, and uterine sarcoma, which arises in the muscular wall of the uterus. It is suggested that women who are taking this drug have regular pelvic examinations and be checked promptly if they have any abnormal vaginal bleeding or pelvic pain. Tamoxifen is generally prescribed as a once-a-day pill for a period of five years.

So, now I had another big decision to make. Just when I thought I was through with all the tough choices, it seemed that I was slammed with another one.

I did a lot of research about the pros and cons of the drug, and discussed it at length with my doctors. I didn't have a problem with the idea of hot flashes, since it seemed that my body was entering premature menopause from the chemo anyway. I was already having my fair share of hot flashes. The idea of the uterine cancer frightened me the most. If I took tamoxifen, would I simply be trading one cancer risk for another?

My oncologist informed me that, while the risk of uterine cancer was certainly to be taken seriously, it was really quite small. Based on my family's history with cancer, it was the breast cancer that I should be most concerned about eradicating. Ultimately, I decided that the benefits outweighed the risks in my particular situation. I filled my first prescription and added a daily dose of tamoxifen to my morning routine.

By June of 1999, nearly a year after my diagnosis, I was ready to have the last step of the reconstruction process — the addition of a nipple and areola. It did make me feel somewhat whole again, but little did I know that it was far from being my last surgery, and even further from allowing me to put it all behind me.

With all the surgeries and treatments completed, something began to happen that I could never have anticipated. I started to miss my treatments. Yes, I missed them! I didn't know what to do with myself anymore. For nearly a year I had actively fought for my life. I had gathered

information, interviewed doctors, undergone operations and chemotherapy treatments. For nearly a year I'd spent my days going from
doctor's offices to labs to hospitals. I'd constantly been examined and
prodded and poked and asked to give my medical history. It was horrible. Or was it?

In all that time I was under the constant observation of the medical
profession. For all those months I felt that if anything were to happen to
me, it would be caught immediately, and that I was doing everything
imaginable to regain my health. I felt like a warrior, fighting for my life.
Now what? Now I felt that I was no longer fighting. That I was just sitting
back and allowing the cancer to rear its ugly head again and that this
time it would take over my life. I had longed for this day since the
whole horrible nightmare began. I had marked my last chemo day on
my calendar at the onset. Now I had reached that goal, and I felt sad!

Reaching Out for Help

I started to slip into a depression. It was as if I was treading water
and every now and then my head would go under. It was getting harder
and harder to stay afloat. I had to do something about it. I had to find a
way to incorporate cancer into my life in a positive way. I couldn't allow
the cancer to manage me; I had to manage it.

I tried a couple of different support groups, to no avail. I was often
the only one in the group trying to be positive and upbeat, and it didn't
help that I also was often the youngest woman there!

In time I found a support group for women with school-age children. It was helpful for a while. One of its members was a woman with
whom I could really relate. Terri had two boys about the same age as
mine, and she had been diagnosed six months before I was. I felt that I
would learn much from her. A few weeks into the session, however, she

came to the meeting with news of a recurrence. That was just too much for me to bear. Here I had been comparing myself to her in every way and now she had a recurrence. I couldn't wait to get out of the room. I didn't want to break down in front of her. She needed us, but I just couldn't be there for her.

After much soul-searching, I decided that I couldn't go back to the support group and I was a bit ashamed of myself for feeling that way. The reason for a support group is to do just that — support one another, but I just wasn't ready to watch someone battle a recurrence when it was one of my biggest fears. I thought it best to leave before we got to know one another any better. Through the grapevine I've heard that Terri is doing well, and I continue to pray for her every night.

So, now what?

While searching through a breast cancer website, I stumbled upon an online breast cancer support group. It is run by a woman who lives in Australia and it has members from all over the world — primarily the U.S. Well, this was just what I needed. I could log on at my convenience and give support to whomever I felt needed it. I was able to sift through the posts that were too negative or self-pitying and respond to those that were more upbeat. It was perfect. I found so much support in this group and so much information. I still log on every day to see how everyone is doing. I rarely post messages, though sometimes I'll respond to someone in need, and it is comforting to know that these wonderful women are there for me if I need them. While my physical self had long since healed, this was the beginning of my emotional healing.

Part III

The Courage
to
Strike Back

Genetic Testing

Now that the decade had ended and a new century had begun, it really was time to move forward. I tried to put the cancer behind me, but it wasn't easy. Each morning when I got dressed I was reminded of what my body had gone through in the past year. And there was always the nagging question of why I had gotten cancer when I was still so young. I kept thinking about all the family members that I had lost to cancer. There just had to be a connection. Maybe genetic testing wasn't such an outlandish idea after all. I decided to take another look at it.

Extensive counseling is provided for anyone considering being tested for an inherited genetic predisposition. I decided to see a genetic counselor to assess my risk factors and make an informed decision about being tested.

At present, BRCA1 and BRCA2 (breast cancer 1 and breast cancer 2) are the two most common genes that have been isolated that are known to increase the risk of breast cancers. When a woman is a carrier of these mutations — BRCA1 or BRCA2 — she has a far greater risk of contracting the disease than the general public does. Of the estimated 5–10 percent of cancers believed to be hereditary, 2–3 percent of these hereditary cancers are predicted to be the result of one of these genes passed down through the generations in a family.

Since I was now seriously considering genetic testing, I spent a far greater amount of time with the genetic counselor than I had the first time we met. She took a full medical history including my experience with breast cancer and my overall health. She considered my eating and exercise habits, as well as my monthly menstrual cycles and age at childbirth. The counselor was trying to determine if there was anything else that may have caused my early-onset breast cancer.

After we delved into my family history with cancer, a family tree was compiled. Circles were drawn for the women in the family and squares for the men. Each person who had been diagnosed with cancer got a black mark added to their box or circle. If they had more than one cancer, they got more than one mark. If the person had passed on, a slash was drawn across their box or circle. It was a frightening illustration of my family's cancer battle. The maternal side of the tree had eight black marks, with four slashes. The paternal side was devoid of any black marks. When I took one look at it, everything became evident.

During our lengthy counseling session we discussed the implications of receiving a positive test. As had been explained to me in the past, the genetic counselor gave me specific percentages of risk associated with each mutant gene. A woman with a BRCA1 or BRCA2 mutation has as much as an 85 percent lifetime risk of developing breast cancer and a 10–45 percent lifetime risk of developing ovarian cancer. This was compared to the 10 percent lifetime risk of breast cancer and 1–2 percent lifetime risk of ovarian cancer in the general population. Mutation carriers with a previous breast cancer have up to a 50 percent risk of contralateral breast cancer (new cancer in the other breast) by age 70.

Since BRCA2 is the gene usually associated with *male* breast cancer, and my uncle had breast cancer, the counselor felt quite strongly that I would be more likely to have that mutation. Males who carry alterations in BRCA2 are estimated to have a 5–10 percent risk for breast cancer. A wider tumor spectrum including cancers of the pancreas, prostate, and colon may also be associated with BRCA2 mutations.

Once again, my mind was in a state of information overload. There was just so much material to process. I was still uncertain if I really needed to know whether or not I was a mutation carrier. My options were still the same — yearly mammograms, monthly breast self-exams, diet and exercise. I had done all these things, and yet I still got the cancer. What else could I possibly do?

Well, in fact there *was* something I could do, I just didn't want to face it. I could remove my other, healthy breast. The harsh reality was that if I proved to be a mutation carrier, I had a 50/50 chance of contracting cancer in that breast. Fifty percent! Were these really the odds I wanted to play?

As our session came to a close, the counselor said something that really struck me and helped make my decision. After looking at my family history, my family tree, and the fact that I was only 38 at my diagnosis, she felt very strongly that my cancer was genetic. In fact, she felt that if it wasn't BRCA1 or BRCA2, it was probably an undiscovered mutation. That really clinched it for me. I would be tested. In fact, I found myself *wanting* to be positive for one of the two known genes. At least scientists had information on these mutations. If I were positive, I could do something about it. I could remove the other breast. It wasn't an idea I relished, but it was something proactive I could do. I just couldn't do it right then. I needed to take some time to collect myself after a year of so many surgeries.

My blood was drawn and sent to the lab. Now all I had to do was wait, something I was getting good at. Still, I needed to feel that I was doing something productive.

Writing as Healing

Having kept a journal since I was 12 years old, I turned to writing. In addition to my personal journal entries, I began writing stories about my experience with breast cancer. I wrote several articles and sent them to various magazines and newspapers. I was pleased when two different articles were picked up by local papers. I was beginning to feel as if I really had something to offer. After all, my breast cancer experience was as positive as it could be. I was blessed to have the love of my husband and children. I had three sisters and my dad, in-laws and good friends. I truly did have everything. There were so many women out there who weren't as blessed as I. Maybe I could help them through it. Perhaps they would like to read about someone who has been there and made it through to the other side.

In response to a request for stories about cancer diagnoses, I submitted an article to New York Newsday. To my surprise and delight, it was published.

The morning that the article ran, before I had even opened my morning newspaper, I received a phone call from a woman I had never met. She'd read my story and found my number in the phone book. She went on to tell me that she was about to begin chemotherapy treatments for breast cancer and was terribly afraid and discouraged. She mentioned that she had just sat down with her cup of tea and the paper to try to forget her troubles when she stumbled across my story. My words had given her hope . . . my words had given her strength. What she didn't realize was that her words did the same for me. It was all beginning to make sense to me now. We could each help one another. Maybe my family history was not such a curse after all. Maybe my knowledge and experience could help someone else. Maybe I should share it in the hope of doing some good.

The essay came out on February 14, 2000 — seventeen years to the day from my mother's death. It also was the day I found out that I carried the BRCA2 mutation.

Journal Entry — Monday, February 14, 2000

My article was published in Newsday *today. I'm both excited and embarrassed. I just wanted to show people that there* **is** *hope. When I write these things it also renews my faith in myself and makes me feel like, yes, in fact, I will be okay.*

I got my results back from the genetic testing today. I do have the BRCA2 mutation. What a surprise (ha). We went over my options, like prophylactic mastectomy, etc. Nothing new. I really don't feel anything at all. I'll just proceed as usual for now.

Reaching Out to Help

One of the defining moments I recall from the first days after my diagnosis was when I called a local breast cancer hotline. While struggling with my first major decision about whether to have a lumpectomy or a mastectomy, I picked up the phone and dialed a number given to me by a friend. The phone was answered and before the woman could even tell me her name, I began rattling off questions. "What do you know about breast cancer?" "What's the difference between lumpectomy and mastectomy?" "How do I know which is right for me?"

The caring soul on the other end of the phone knew exactly what I was going through. Her response was kind and calming. The first thing she said was, "Take a deep breath and slow down for a second. First let me tell you that my name is Barbara, and I am a breast cancer survivor."

Suddenly the tears began to flow. I hadn't given myself a moment to cry until then. The tears just came and came and I could barely speak. Between sobs, I managed to muster a garbled "I'm sorry . . . I'm sorry, I haven't even cried yet."

Barbara turned out to be yet another angel in my nightmare. She was very knowledgeable, and she lovingly shared her own experience with me. We chatted for a while and she mailed me some pertinent information. The best part of it all was that she had been there and was still around to talk about it! If this kind, faceless person on the other end of the phone could survive, maybe I would as well.

The Hotline

I thought of Barbara when I learned that the Adelphi NY Statewide Breast Cancer Hotline & Support Program was looking for volunteers. The program is located at Adelphi University, about 30 minutes from my home. Volunteers were needed to work on the hotline and do neighborhood outreaches. *Perhaps I could be someone's "Barbara."* I picked up the phone and dialed their number.

I began training as a volunteer in the spring of 2000. The program's mission is to educate, support, empower and advocate for breast cancer patients, their families and the community. The training consisted of six two-hour sessions conducted by a certified social worker. There were about 20 women in my training class, most of whom were breast cancer survivors. Each week a new topic was discussed and a new expert was invited to speak. We each shared our own experiences so that we might learn from one another. We even did role playing, pretending to be callers with various questions and concerns.

The breast cancer hotline is a large part of Adelphi's mission, but they do far more than that. They provide information to the community on all aspects of breast cancer. Forums on breast health and new technologies are provided as the need arises. Support groups are offered by trained social workers and targeted at specific situations such as *women with young children* or *newly diagnosed women.* They even offer a support group for spouses. Everything is confidential and free of charge.

Each and every staff member was invited to our training class to introduce themselves and tell us about their role. We were trained on how to answer the phone and how to allay other women's fears. The staff was always available to help out if any of us received a particularly difficult call or one where we felt the caller needed more professional help. It was the most caring, loving, heartwarming atmosphere I had ever experienced. I immediately felt as if I belonged. This was where I wanted to be and what I wanted to do. I had found my niche!

When my training was complete, I began working on the breast cancer hotline. Each time I answer the phone I encounter a new and different situation. Sometimes I feel that I wasn't helpful at all, but usually it is just the opposite. There is nothing that can compare with knowing you just calmed someone's fears and helped them to see that there is light at the end of the tunnel.

In addition to the hotline I also work at some outreaches. An outreach is any community event that helps educate about breast cancer. Organizers of a health fair may ask Adelphi to provide a table with some information. Or perhaps a women's group may want a speaker. I've even done outreaches as simple as wrapping gifts at a bookstore. At every outreach there is always someone who really needs our help and learns something about her own health by our presence. We have a lot to offer the community, and I am more than happy to be one of the messengers. I try to avail myself of as many outreaches as possible. It is always a mutually beneficial experience.

So now it seemed as if I was putting the horror of the cancer behind me and incorporating the positive aspects of it into my life. I felt healthy, alive and active. Nearly two years had passed since that horrible phone call shattered my innocence. Life was good again. My children were growing up happy and healthy, and now it looked as if they would have their mom around for a while. My relationship with Jay was better than ever; the cancer only made us stronger. I wanted to shout out to the world, "I survived! I'm a breast cancer survivor!" I wanted to celebrate. So when I heard about the Avon Breast Cancer 3-Day, it seemed as if I could do just that and raise money and awareness at the same time.

Avon Breast Cancer 3-Day

The Avon Breast Cancer 3-Day was a 60-mile walk sponsored by Avon to raise funds for breast cancer research. The walks were held in various parts of the country and spanned three days. Each person agreed to raise a minimum of $1,800 to support national nonprofit breast health programs and medical research on women's diseases.

The 2000 New York event began at Bear Mountain State Park in upstate New York and ended in Manhattan. Over 3,000 participants spent three days walking approximately 20 miles a day and two nights camped out in a makeshift "tent city." The sponsors provided the tents, three meals a day, "pit stops" for drinks and snacks, Porta Potties, and even entertainment. Walkers provided their own sleeping bags and other camping gear, which would be moved along the route in gear trucks manned by volunteer crew members. It was being billed as "three days that will change your life."

Wow, this was something I had to do! It screamed out to me. After all, I worked in Avon's corporate offices for over 10 years and was even the co-captain of Avon's team for the Corporate Challenge — a 3-mile foot race in Central Park. I was avidly interested in fitness and exercise, and I was a breast cancer survivor. The Avon 3-Day was created for **me.** I just had to do it. But could I? Could I really walk 60 miles? And what about sleeping in a tent? I was not really one for sleeping in the great outdoors; I needed plumbing and electricity! No matter. Somehow I would make it work. I would complete the Avon Breast Cancer 3-Day if it was the last thing I did!

The New York walk was scheduled for the weekend of October 13–15. October 15th was my 41st birthday — another sign that this walk was made for me! I sent away for the packet of information and began talking to family and friends about the event. When all three of my sisters signed on to do the walk along with me, it was the icing on the cake. Now I knew it was going to be great. How ideal to have four sisters with such a strong family history of cancer be a part of the fight for a cure!

Once the 3-Day packet arrived in the mail my anxiety was replaced by excitement and anticipation. I could barely talk or think about anything else. While Avon sponsored the event, it was run by a company called Pallotta Teamworks. Pallotta organized the event so well that nothing was left to chance. We were given pointers on fundraising, training, what to wear and pack, and even where to buy the proper sneakers. Once we registered, we were sent monthly newsletters that updated us on the status of other 3-Days around the country and counted down the days to the New York event. We received profiles on some of the walkers and lists of those who would be walking in our area. Now all I had to do was train!

Although I had been exercising regularly for years, proper training in *walking* was strongly suggested, so I began training in late March. I started out with some three and four-mile walks in my neighborhood, soon realizing that much more mileage was required for me to get in the proper shape for the event. None of my sisters lived in my neighborhood and I was starting to get nervous about being able to do so much training alone. Then I got an e-mail from a walker in my area looking for a training partner. We decided to meet at a local park for an early morning walk. I was skeptical at first — after all, I was meeting a total stranger in a deserted park — but our meeting turned out to be just what I needed.

Diane D. was participating in the Avon 3-Day alone. She was walking for her aunt, who had breast cancer. She introduced me to Lisa, whom she had also met through an e-mail. The three of us began training together and we became fast friends. We talked about everything — our husbands, jobs, kids and in-laws. We talked about our reasons for walking and our excitement over receiving another check toward our goal. During each of our training walks there was always something new to share. We continued to spread the word to other walkers in surrounding areas and before we knew it, our little group had expanded. On any given Saturday or Sunday morning you could be sure to have several people to train with and to share another story of hope and survival.

There was Karen, walking in memory of her mom, who died of breast cancer when her first child was just 6 months old; Carey, walking in memory of her aunt and in support of her friend Mary, who was walking along with her; Naomi, a very hip, in-shape grandmother walking to honor the memory of her first cousin, who died from breast cancer while pregnant with her second child; Diane C., also walking in memory of a cousin; Carol W., in memory of her sister-in-law and in support of several friends; Susan, Nancy, Elyse, Carole L., Samantha, Christine . . . the list goes on and on. Each of these remarkable women joined in the fight for the most selfless of reasons — to help find a cure for a disease that has destroyed the lives of so many innocent women (and men).

We walked throughout the spring and into summer. The training I initially dreaded turned into something I really looked forward to. With each predawn drive to the park to meet my walking buddies, I felt happier, more alive and secure in the fact that I now had firmly moved from a victim to a survivor. And while our bodies got stronger and more in shape, our hearts became full and nurtured by the outpouring of love and compassion shared with one another. Since I was getting such pleasure out of the training, I could barely imagine what the actual event would be like!

There was one part of this event, however, that I did not relish — fundraising. I didn't know how I would be able to raise $1,800, especially since all three of my sisters were walking with me. I certainly couldn't expect family members to donate to all four of us. That's when I decided to do a letter-writing campaign. I wrote from my heart, describing the effect that breast cancer has had on my entire family, including my own personal experience. I mentioned all those who had lost the battle and stressed the importance of striving to raise awareness so that we can put an end to this horrendous disease.

The money came pouring in. Within the first month I received around $600. My friends and family reached deep into their pockets to donate to a cause that was so close to my heart and had touched me so personally. I especially enjoyed the notes and phone calls I received along with some of the donations. Many wrote that they, too, had been affected by breast cancer and they applauded our efforts to try to help eradicate this terrible disease. In no time at all I had surpassed my goal of $1,800. By the time the walk took place, my fundraising efforts had topped out at just over $7,500; adding it together with all three sisters' donations it was over $20,000. I was dumbfounded by the generosity of people.

By the end of September the training had really paid off — my body was fit and ready. My donations were in, gear was purchased and bags were packed. All that was left was the event itself. I was so excited that I could barely contain myself! Now we just had to hope for the weather to cooperate.

Journal Entry — Wednesday, October 11, 2000
It's the night before the walk and I'm very excited. The weather is supposed to be beautiful. I can't wait! I hope to write in here while I'm gone.

The walk would begin on Friday, but we were required to meet at Bear Mountain on Thursday for what was being called "Day Zero." We rode the bus with other walkers from Long Island and Queens. When we arrived at Bear Mountain, it was as if a small city had been constructed just for us. There were tents set up everywhere, labeled "registration," "tent assignments," "safety video," "medical," etc. It was all very organized, and everyone was friendly and happy to be there. It had finally arrived! I was finally on the 3-Day!

After registering and receiving our tent assignments, we went on to see the required safety video. Then we headed back to our hotel to check in and walked across the street for dinner, where the restaurant was filled with the excitement and bustle of hundreds of walkers! We chatted eagerly with some new friends as we dined. We were in bed by 9:00 p.m. in preparation for our early morning excursion, which would have a profound effect on the rest of my life.

Our journey began in the predawn hours of Friday, October 13, 2000. The sun was rising and the weather magnificent as the opening ceremonies began. Dan Pallotta, the president of Pallotta Teamworks, spoke eloquently about the event ahead of us. He commended us for being there and taking on such a huge adventure, calling us "heroes" and comparing us to the likes of Rosa Parks and John F. Kennedy! I certainly didn't feel like a hero. I hadn't even done anything yet!

Then we listened to several survivors briefly tell their stories of hope before joining their hands to form a circle. They proceeded off the stage and down a path created by hundreds of walkers on either side. As the human circle marched on, a speaker was explaining the meaning of it all. The outside of the circle celebrated life and hope, while the empty center was the memory of all those lost to this dreadful disease. Beautiful music was playing, the sun was peeking over the mountain, and the birds were singing. It couldn't have been staged any more beautifully if it had been on a movie lot in Hollywood. There was not a dry eye in the bunch! Suddenly the music got louder, the horn sounded, and the 2000 Avon Breast Cancer 3-Day officially began.

Journal Entry — Friday, October 13, 2000

I'm in my tent now on the 3-Day. This has been the most amazing day and a half of my life. I really don't have the words to express it. The weather is absolutely perfect. We are walking with the women we trained with, and it is making the whole experience so much nicer. We are having a ball. All four of us sisters stayed together today. We also met some new people.

Oops . . . it's getting too dark now and it's "lights out" soon, so I'd better go.

For the next three days we traded our warm beds, flushable toilets and long hot showers for sleeping bags, Porta Potties and shower trucks. We walked past churches and schools, through towns and parks. We walked, walked, walked . . . and then we walked some more! Each street was a new adventure. The one thing each place had in common was the number of people who came out to support our efforts.

There were the uniformed schoolchildren on the side of the road cheering us on. And the Girl Scouts pinning star stickers on us while chanting, "You're a star." A local high school marching band played

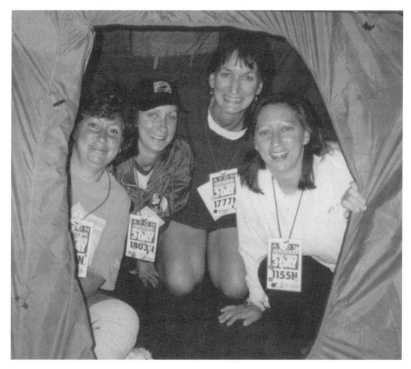

Avon 3-Day Walk — October 2000. My sisters and I cozy up in our tent. Left to right: Linda, Laura, Me, Carol.

while their cheerleaders, pom-poms in hand, jumped, tumbled and belted out their approval. Even the local bakery was out in force, offering pink ribbon–shaped cookies they had baked in our honor. It was a truly remarkable outpouring of support.

Along our journey we were guided by the all-volunteer crew, which rode beside us on bicycles, motorcycles and in vans to motivate us and keep us safe. They shouted encouragement through bullhorns, telling us how many miles were behind and how many more ahead.

Every few miles we arrived at a pit stop, where we could get drinks and snacks and use the Porta Potti. Since safety was their first concern, the crew would gently advise us at each pit stop to "hydrate and urinate" because "if you don't pee, you'll get an IV."

With each step we took another story was told. We met a man who was walking in honor of his mother and sister. He had purchased 300 small American flags to give out along the route. There was an older gentleman walking with a cane — slowly, one step at a time. Then there was the 24-year-old woman with metastasized breast cancer. This was her second 3-Day event. She tore her Achilles tendon and dehydrated on Saturday. She spent the night in the hospital and came back on crutches to complete the walk with us on Sunday.

At camp each night, the crew provided us with abundant meals (I gained two pounds!) and entertainment. It was "lights out" at 9:00 p.m., when I discovered that a sleeping bag never felt so good. We awoke to another glorious day on Saturday, and again on Sunday.

To get from New Jersey to Manhattan on Sunday, we were to walk over the George Washington Bridge. Throughout all of our training, this was what we had all been anticipating. It was the symbol that we had actually completed this momentous task and were now arriving at the closing ceremonies. I will never forget the euphoria I felt as we crossed the bridge on foot. The arduous tasks of fundraising and training were behind me now. All the excitement I had felt (albeit laced with moments of self-doubt) was finally coming to fruition. We had completed the Avon Breast Cancer 3-Day! I couldn't wait to see my family and friends. With blistered feet and sore muscles, we entered Manhattan's Morningside Park to a scene more moving than I could ever have imagined.

Before the closing ceremonies, all the walkers gathered in a common area as everyone was accounted for. While we waited for one another, we were all given T-shirts — blue ones to the "regular" walkers, pink ones to the "survivors." Those with blue T-shirts gathered behind a large curtain until the speaker announced that the walkers had arrived. At that point the curtain was pulled aside to reveal the hundreds and hundreds of family members and friends who had come to welcome us home. There were barricades on either side of the path left open for the walkers. People were cheering, crying and waving banners as the walkers processed down the path leading them to their loved ones.

My sisters had already gone in with the rest. I was still behind the curtain with the other pink-clad survivors until it was time for us to be announced. When the curtain was pulled aside again, we were led through the same path, now narrowed by our fellow walkers. Again, everyone was cheering and crying — not out of sadness, but from the sheer joy of having completed such a task. I was desperately searching the faces in the crowd for Jay and our kids. Finally, I spotted them. There they were, holding a huge banner welcoming us home. Each of my sons had made his own sign as well, congratulating me and wishing me a happy birthday. The families of all three of my sisters were there too, along with my dad, Aunt Fran, two cousins and some friends.

The survivors joined together with the other walkers while the curtain was pulled aside one last time, ushering in the all-volunteer

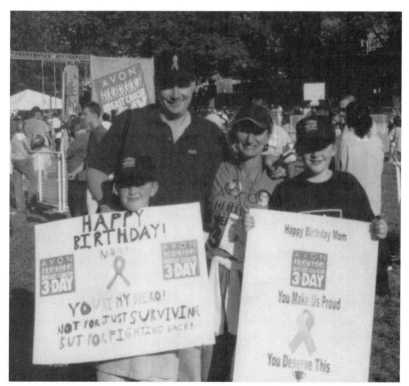

Conclusion of the Avon 3-Day Walk. Jay and me with our kids.

crew. They arrived to thunderous applause and cheers as we shouted out our thanks for their tireless efforts to keep us safe, hydrated and very, very well fed. After some brief speeches, the crowd dispersed and we all traveled home with our loved ones, each of us richer for having shared such a life-affirming experience. My 41st birthday is one I will never forget!

Shortly afterward, I signed up for the 2001 event.

Proactive Defense

After experiencing the ultimate satisfaction in completing my goal of finishing the walk, the new year arrived with its own set of fresh decisions and challenges. Being shy of two years since my diagnosis, and knowing my genetic status; I still felt that I had many decisions to make regarding my health, and that I was far from "out of the woods." So early in the year I went to see my gynecologist.

Ovaries

After determining that I was, in fact, in chemo-induced early meno-pause, I made the decision to have my healthy ovaries removed in a procedure called a "prophylactic oophorectomy." Out came my green notebook, and a new section added — *oophorectomy*. As health decisions go, this one was fairly simple. My ovaries were no longer viable, and the procedure was not terribly invasive or painful. Being in menopause possibly a decade earlier than I should was no picnic, but the chemo had already taken care of that. Removing my ovaries at this point in my life would not change anything other than the fact that I would no longer have to worry about ovarian cancer. My BRCA2 status put my risk of developing ovarian cancer possibly as high as 25 percent, as opposed to a 1–2 percent chance for the general population. Yes, this seemed like a decision I just had to make.

I had the prophylactic oophorectomy in March 2001. We arrived at the hospital early in the morning for the pre-op procedures. I was very nervous as they hooked me up to the IV and took my blood pressure and medical history again. As the hours ticked away with no further activity, I began to get agitated and cranky. All of a sudden a strikingly attractive man entered the room and introduced himself as my anesthesiologist. He asked me a whole new line of questions and then was called away for a minute. Jay turned to me and said, "Is it just me, or is he very good-looking?" "Oh my God, you noticed too?" I replied. With that, Dr. Tall, Dark and Handsome returned with one of the nurses. As he continued to question me, the nurse was practically tripping over herself and giggling like a schoolgirl. Jay and I could no longer look at each other without bursting into laughter. Once again, our good humor got us through!

The oophorectomy was performed laparoscopically on an outpatient basis, and I was home that same night. When I awoke I was surprised to find only three Band-Aids marking the locations where the procedure was done, one over my navel and one over the spot where each ovary had been. It didn't seem like enough. I mean, these were my ovaries, the organ that produced my first period as a teen and fed my body estrogen all my life. The organ that released the eggs that became my two beautiful children. I felt there should have been more drama. I had gone to sleep and when I woke up my ovaries were gone and all I had to show for them was three Band-Aids! It was simple — physically, but emotionally, I did mourn my ovaries for a while. Eventually, I realized that my "womanhood" was no more dependant upon my ovaries than it was on my breasts. Ultimately, what matters is my good health and long life so I can be here for my children.

Journal Entry — Saturday, March 3, 2001

I'm sitting in my favorite recliner with the comforter on my lap, recovering from my oophorectomy, which I had on Thursday. All went well and I feel pretty good. Just very sore and even my shoulders hurt from the gas, but not really too much to complain about. I'm still taking painkillers every 4 hours, but I am definitely getting better every day. I slept really well last night, but woke up pretty uncomfortable. It subsided as the day wore on and I am so happy that it is finally over . . .

Journal Entry — Friday, March 9, 2001

Wednesday was my first day out and boy was I ever ready to get out! Met some friends for lunch and did a little grocery shopping. Yesterday I went in to Adelphi to work the hotline. The staff gave me flowers to welcome me back. It was very busy but, odd as it sounds, I really feel so alive when I am there.

As soon as I got home I needed to get back into my sweats, though. My stomach is still a bit sore. I'll wait until after the weekend to put my jeans back on.

Laura's Decision

Right around the time that I was finally feeling comfortable that I had made sound decisions about my health, my sister Laura was struggling with her own demons regarding her health. All three of my sisters had genetic testing after my cancer diagnosis. Both Linda and Laura are BRCA2 positive and are tormented by the same fears of cancer that I am. Thankfully, Carol tested negative.

Having had a hysterectomy three years earlier, Linda was free from the ovarian cancer scare, but still very worried about breast cancer. She has since become very proactive in her screening — undergoing MRIs, ultrasounds and mammograms, in addition to her clinical breast exams and monthly self-exams. Additionally, Linda chose to go on a five-year course of tamoxifen to further reduce her risk of being stricken with the disease. In clinical trials tamoxifen has been shown to lower breast cancer risk by as much as 50 percent, although the level of risk reduction is not as well studied for women with gene mutations.

Linda was feeling confident that she was an active participant in her own well-being, though there may come a day, she has stated, when she will decide to undergo prophylactic mastectomies.

Conversely, at this point in time Laura was trying to decide whether or not to have a bilateral prophylactic mastectomy. She'd had many, many lumps — all thankfully benign — and numerous breast surgeries. But Laura was beginning to feel that she was running out of luck. Although it is impossible to remove every bit of breast tissue during a mastectomy, the procedure still significantly reduces the risk of breast cancer.

My sister began looking into different kinds of reconstructive surgeries before making her final decision. Since she wasn't dealing with a cancer, she was able to take her time and research as many different possibilities as were available.

There are several kinds of breast reconstruction available today. The two most widely used are implant reconstruction, which is what I had, and TRAM flap reconstruction. TRAM flap reconstruction involves the movement of tissues (skin, underlying fatty tissues, and muscle) from the abdomen to create a new breast. When this type of procedure is done, patients are left with a long scar across the abdomen that is very similar to the scar left by a cosmetic abdominoplasty ("tummy tuck") with the abdominal wall nicely recontoured.

There are several advantages to this type of reconstruction. Since TRAM flap involves using your own tissue, the risk of infection is lower and it is also typically easier to match the contralateral natural breast. A TRAM flap generally yields a rather natural-looking breast and there is no worry of having "foreign material" left inside the chest wall, as there is with implant reconstruction.

Although TRAMs are highly successful and still a very good option for many patients, there are a few disadvantages as well. Because the abdominal muscles are cut and a portion removed, patients are left with some abdominal wall weakness. They are also at increased risk for abdominal wall hernias. Much of the discomfort many patients feel after this type of surgery is not in the area of the new breast, but rather in the abdomen, where the muscles were cut.

The implant reconstruction that I had is a much easier procedure. Like the TRAM flap, it is typically started at the same time as the mastectomy, but unlike the TRAM flap, it requires two to three separate surgeries to complete. A temporary implant, called an expander, is placed under the pectoral muscle at the time of the mastectomy. The expander is filled each week to stretch the tissues gradually. A second surgery is required to remove the expander and replace it with the final implant. The nipple and areola are added during a third surgery.

The obvious disadvantage to this type of reconstruction is the need for three separate surgeries, each requiring general anesthesia. Additionally, several problems can occur due to the fact that the implant is left under the skin indefinitely. Some women may feel discomfort or tightness in the breast area. Moreover, after ten or more years, the chance of implant rupture is great, necessitating another surgery to replace it.

There are many advantages to this type of surgery as well. Implant reconstruction is a relatively simple procedure. While it does require repeated surgeries, none are terribly painful or require a long recovery period. It does not cause any additional scarring and, more importantly, it does not compromise the abdominal muscle wall.

When I was making my decision regarding reconstruction, I was in the throes of trying to sort out and deal with the fact that I had cancer. There were still so many unknowns: Would my nodes be positive? Would I be required to have radiation? Chemotherapy? Would I even live long enough to care if I had breasts at all?

As with all my other health decisions, I consulted two plastic surgeons before choosing my reconstruction method. Although I liked the idea of using my own tissue (TRAM flap), the length of surgery and weeks of recovery frightened me terribly. And, being very active, I wasn't pleased about compromising my abdominal muscles. After my two consults the decision was made for me. Both doctors felt that I didn't have enough abdominal fat to form an adequate-sized breast. At best, they felt they could possibly construct *one* small breast, but if the need ever arose for me to remove the other breast, there was definitely not enough fat to construct two. I felt relieved. I had so much to deal with regarding the cancer alone, I surely didn't need to be adding such a painful surgery into the mix.

Laura, on the other hand, had a much different perspective. She had struggled with the decision to have a bilateral prophylactic mastectomy for so long. Since there was no cancer involved, she was willing to undergo a more invasive surgery to ensure a good result.

While Laura researched her options, I started to have doubts about my choices. Since she was so adamant about *not* having the implant reconstruction that I had opted for, I began to take another look at my body. Was my reconstruction so terrible? Did my breast not look natural? Why in the world was this an option she was so dead-set against?

I was surprised to find myself having these body image problems three years after my reconstruction, and I despised the fact that I had so many feelings of self-doubt. After all, I had made the best decision I could at the time, based on my individual situation!

After beating myself up about feeling that way, I came to realize that maybe this was a good sign. A healthy dose of vanity was a symbol that I had come far from just worrying about whether I was going to live or die. Now that I realized I was going to *live*, I wanted to *look* good too.

After hours in front of the mirror scrutinizing my body, I came to terms with all of my decisions regarding my reconstruction. What bothered me the most was the fact that my breasts were not symmetrical. Two pregnancies and nine months of breast feeding had taken a toll on my natural breast. My implant was "perky" and I was self-conscious that others could tell that my breasts didn't "match" exactly. In the end, though, I felt quite certain that the day would come when I would remove my natural breast since I had up to a 50 percent chance of contracting cancer on that side. It was just not something I was ready to do at this point. I had already had seven surgeries in the past three years and I needed a break! Somewhere down the line I would find the strength to endure another mastectomy, but now it was Laura's turn. I would support her in her decision.

Through all her research, Laura had stumbled upon another type of new reconstruction that I had never heard of. It was called DIEP flap.

Journal Entry — March 5, 2001

Laura found a doctor on Long Island who does a special kind of new surgery that doesn't use the muscle. It's called DIEP flap. I hope she's making the right decision. A part of me is a little jealous since I know her breasts are going to look so much better than mine. What the hell is wrong with me? This isn't a beauty contest and I wouldn't have had a larger surgery anyway! I hate myself when I have these horrible feelings. It is such a big surgery, though, and I hope she realizes what she's in for.

DIEP flap breast reconstruction was relatively new when Laura heard about it in 2001. This type of surgery is similar to TRAM flap reconstruction in that it also uses tissues taken from the abdomen. One major difference, however, is that the DIEP flap is a microsurgical technique and does not use the abdominal muscle.

Like the TRAM flap procedure, DIEP flap involves moving of tissues from the abdomen to construct a new breast. The major difference in a DIEP flap procedure is that the flap is actually detached and the blood vessels reattached to blood vessels under the breastbone (internal mammary vessels.) Microsurgery is used to isolate the blood vessels and sew the small vessels together with very fine sutures and instruments. Less of the muscle is used since the flap is healthier and has a better blood supply.

The obvious advantages to this type of surgery are essentially the same as with the TRAM flap. It has a lower risk of infection because of the use of one's own tissue, and it does not introduce any foreign material into the body.

Since the muscle is left intact, there is much less risk of abdominal wall weakness and hernia. In addition, there is clearly less discomfort following DIEP surgery than following TRAM surgery. Because of the reduced pain and the fact that the muscle wall remains intact, patients are often able to get back to their normal daily routines more quickly.

As with any surgical procedure, there are disadvantages to a DIEP flap as well. Because it is a more complex procedure involving micro-surgery, it takes a great deal longer, necessitating a longer time under anesthesia and a longer hospital stay. Women are left with both a breast scar and an abdominal scar. And, while the recuperation is easier than with the TRAM flap, it is still substantially longer than with implant reconstruction.

After Laura carefully weighed all her options, she finally decided upon the DIEP flap procedure. It was a far more complex reconstructive surgery than the implant surgery that I'd had. Since she would require blood transfusions, Laura donated some of her own blood prior to the surgery and family members volunteered to donate their blood for her as well.

Laura entered the hospital in April 2001. Her mastectomies and DIEP flap procedure took 16 hours to complete, while the doctor dissected and then reattached major blood vessels from her abdomen to form two new breasts. We all waited nervously at home until we received the phone call that her surgery was finally completed.

Journal Entry — Wednesday, April 18, 2001
Laura's surgery was yesterday at 7 a.m. She didn't come out until 11:15 p.m.!
I was really nervous and very anxious for her all day.

She remained in the hospital for nearly a week as she recovered. Her pain was minimal, but she had drains not only in the areas of her breasts but in the groin area as well. Slowly Laura regained her strength. She returned to the hospital several months later to have the nipple and areola reconstructed. When it was all completed, Laura was very happy with her results. More importantly, she would no longer have to go through the terrifying experience of having biopsy after biopsy each and every time she saw her breast surgeon. She would still live with the fear of ovarian cancer but at this point in time Laura decided to leave her ovaries intact.

Life moved forward without incident, but this time for only a few months.

Round Two

At my insistence, early in the summer of 2001 my doctor prescribed a screening MRI on my remaining breast. Her reluctance was due to the fact that MRIs depict many microscopic abnormalities, many too small to biopsy, and often benign. Therefore, this procedure often causes undue anxiety. I felt that this was a small price to pay for the peace of mind I would feel if the results were normal. And if they weren't normal, this procedure would be the catalyst I needed to finally remove my remaining breast.

The MRI uncovered two small "spots" on my breast. As my doctor predicted, a needle biopsy proved inconclusive since the radiologist wasn't even sure that she'd targeted the correct spots. Again I had new information that I needed to digest. There were two abnormalities which the doctors felt were *probably* benign, but *could* be malignant — and ultimately fatal if left to grow.

Journal Entry — Saturday, July 14, 2001

I got my MRI results and they saw two spots, 3 mm each. I had a mammo and sonogram and they could only find one spot, which they think is probably a cyst. Now they'll try to aspirate it. If that doesn't work, they'll try a core biopsy. Bottom line — I'm going to have a mastectomy no matter what the outcome. I always knew I'd have the other breast removed, but wasn't sure when. Well, this just made my decision for me.

Tuesday night I barely slept at all. Right now I am fine with everything, but bottom line — I'm terrified! I was crying at the radiology lab.

It was the 3-year anniversary of my diagnosis too! It was as if nothing had ever changed and I was thrown right back to the brink of depression again.

Well, if ever there was a sign to have a prophylactic mastectomy, this was it. Here we go again. I dusted off my green notebook, added a section entitled round two and braced myself for three more surgeries! This time I felt much more in control. There was no rush to get it done since, as far as we knew, there was no cancer to worry about. Having switched insurance companies over the previous three years, I was now forced to find a new breast surgeon. She came highly recommended and I was beginning to have a relationship with her, so I felt pretty confident. I would use the same plastic surgeon since I held him in high regard. Now all that was left was scheduling, right? Wrong!

My breast surgeon was the first one to throw a wrench into the mix. Usually when a prophylactic mastectomy is performed, the lymph nodes under the arm are left intact. With no reason to believe that cancer is present, there is no reason to remove the nodes. Lymph nodes are needed to drain fluid from that area, when they are removed, problems can arise.

With the sentinel node biopsy I had the first time around, only nine lymph nodes had been removed. Still, it was recommended that I treat that arm carefully, that I not have blood drawn or blood pressure taken on that arm.

My surgeon was now informing me that new studies suggested a sentinel node biopsy even during a prophylactic mastectomy. Now what? Should I allow her to remove lymph nodes from my other arm, leaving myself prone to further problems in the future? I didn't take this decision lightly.

If we did the sentinel node procedure, radioactive material and blue dye would be injected under the nipple prior to the surgery. Lymph nodes that became radioactive or blue would be removed. Most of the time one lymph node picks up both tracers, so only a single lymph node is removed.

If I chose not to have this procedure done and my breast tissue was malignant, they would have to remove all the lymph nodes, in the absence of a breast in which to inject the dye. That would be the only way to determine if the cancer had spread. It would also put me at a much greater risk of developing lymphedema in the future. Once again, I was feeling as if I didn't have much choice. My doctor assured me that the removal of one or two nodes should not affect the drainage of fluid and I should not expect to have any problems with lymphedema in the future.

While I was still struggling with that decision, my plastic surgeon threw me another curve ball. In the time that had transpired since my first implant reconstruction, silicone implants had now been FDA approved for breast reconstruction in breast cancer patients. My doctor felt rather strongly that a silicone implant would yield a more natural result than the saline implant I currently had. My excitement was quickly replaced with trepidation once I began reading the material he gave me from the Institute of Medicine (IOM).

Until the 1990s, most implants contained a synthetic silicone gel that often had a more pleasing feel and look than today's saline-filled implants. But this same silicone gel has caused controversy because of fears that it can potentially produce ill effects in women receiving breast implants. Some women allege that the silicone in implants, particularly the silicone gel inside the implant sac, can cause connective tissue or other autoimmune diseases such as rheumatoid arthritis and lupus, neurological disorders and even cancer. As a result of this belief, many lawsuits were filed against implant manufacturers by women claiming they were harmed by silicone breast implants.

In 1992 the FDA banned most uses of silicone-filled implants because the manufacturers had not proved their safety. In 1993, the agency notified saline implant manufacturers that they, too, must submit safety and effectiveness data, although these implants were allowed to stay on the market. An IOM committee study and report subsequently ensued, and in 2001 silicone gel implants were again a viable choice for implant reconstruction. There was a lot more to consider than just how I was going to look.

In reading the study closely, I discovered that silicone is derived from silica, the most common substance on earth. Silicone can be found in many common household items such as suntan lotion, soaps, and chewing gum. In fact, even saline-filled implants are encased in a silicone shell.

Decisions, decisions, decisions! Oh, how I hated making all these difficult decisions. It seemed that every time I felt that my life was back on track, something would occur to make me doubt myself again. I was frantically trying to gather information on both the sentinel node procedure and silicone implants when it happened. For the second time in this whole nightmare something occurred that forced me to see the bigger picture. In 1998, when I was first dealing with my cancer, Sarah's tragic and untimely death brought me back to reality. And now, in the fall of 2001, the most horrific and terrifying event, beyond anyone's imagination, would take my thoughts away from myself and show me just how insignificant my problems were in the larger scheme of things.

September 11, 2001

It was around 9:00 a.m. when my telephone rang. Barbara, my mother-in-law, told me to turn on the television: apparently a plane had crashed into the World Trade Center. I switched on the TV and watched as the tower billowed smoke and flames. Initially, I thought it was just a deadly pilot error. As I stood there in disbelief another plane crashed into the second tower. Oh, my God! This couldn't be a mistake. This is an attack! I dialed Jay's work number at Two World Trade Center. The call didn't go through.

North tower, south tower . . . the newscasters were rambling on about which tower had been hit first and which one hit second. I had no idea which tower Jay worked in. I had never heard them referred to as north and south towers. All I knew was that his office was in the World Trade Center. Why didn't the telephone calls go through? I needed to talk to Jay!

After a second or two, my mind began to clear. Wait a minute...Jay wasn't in the city today! He was out of the country on business. That's right; he was on another business trip. One of those damn trips that took him away from the kids and me all too many times. One of those trips that both he and I dreaded. One of those trips that may have saved his life!

I tried to pull myself together long enough to drive Brian to school. When he got out of the car he said, "Well, at least this means Daddy will be home for a day or two while they repair his building." I choked back my tears and kissed him goodbye. Neither of us had any idea of the magnitude of destruction that would occur that day.

Once home again, I returned to the television set, as did everyone else as the shocking news began to spread. A short time later my phone began to ring. Family and friends were calling me to inquire about Jay. "He's safe," I would tell them. "He wasn't in the building today." Each time I said the words I became acutely more aware of the terror he had been spared. And though I knew he was safe in Monte Carlo, I still hadn't spoken to him. I really needed to hear his voice.

It was several hours before Jay was able to get through to the United States. He and his colleagues were holed up in a hotel room watching the drama unfold. They still had no idea which floors had been hit, who had made it out safely, and who wasn't as lucky. As we talked on the phone, several calls clicked in through my call waiting. Many of Jay's coworkers were calling him at home to let him know they were safe and to inquire about the others. I fielded the calls and listened to each terrifying story as I switched back and forth between each new caller and Jay. One by one we would account for every person in his department. With a few tragic exceptions, most of the people Jay knew made it out alive on that infamous day.

Content in the knowledge that Jay was safe, I continued to watch in horror and disbelief with the rest of the world as the flames engulfed and ultimately felled the two towers. Selfishly, I marveled again at my own good fortune. While I cried for those who were watching their loved ones perish in front of their eyes, my tears were also shed in gratitude that my family was spared the horror.

I spent some time on the phone with my breast surgeon that afternoon trying to decide on the next steps to be taken for my own well-being and continued health. It all just seemed so insignificant. What was the big deal about losing another breast? What was the big deal about having had cancer? Silicone? Saline? Nothing seemed to matter in the greater scheme of things. How could I ever complain about the misfortunes in my life when so many innocent lives were lost in the most horrendous manner imaginable!

Yes, I would take off the other breast. Yes, I would have to endure three more surgeries. And yes, I would live to see another day. I would live to see many more days. I said a silent prayer and vowed to never again complain about such trivial things.

It was four days before Jay was able to get a flight back home to the U.S. It was with relief and guilt that the kids and I welcomed him home. We were together again as a family, relatively untouched by the catastrophic events that had shattered so many innocent lives. Were we lucky or were we blessed? I think it was a little of both!

Being in Marketing and Communications, Jay returned to New York City the very next day after arriving home. He was responsible for helping set up an interim office, for drafting letters to the victims' families, and for composing communications to the survivors. Yes, they were being referred to as *survivors*. But Jay didn't think he was a survivor.

Of course, he was a survivor. Why should I be the only one? The whole building went down! He could have been there . . . easily. He *should* have been there. But he wasn't. That makes him a survivor. But he doesn't like the word. Maybe because he would have to give in to the enormity of what happened and the fact that it could have happened to him. I'm the one who's supposed to die — not him! Why wasn't he there? Is it fair that we don't have to go through the horror and pain that so many other families are going through? That doesn't seem right.

Yet I'm certainly not asking for the pain. I surely don't want the pain. I guess I just want reasons. And not one of us has reasons.

So many innocent people lost their lives that day. I keep imagining the terror. The terror of the people on the planes. The terror of the people in their offices, just starting their day. Maybe drinking their morning coffee or catching up with a coworker. Then all of a sudden… that's it — it's over. Life is gone in a split second!

What of all those left behind? The innocent people whose lives have been shattered, not just by the loss of their loved ones but by the knowledge of how they were lost. And by the pain they may have felt. And the fear. My God, the fear!

Of course he is a survivor! He worked on the 53rd floor. He should have been there. But he wasn't. He wasn't. Thank God, he wasn't!

Everything else seems rather insignificant now — the breast cancer, the surgeries, the chemo. I'm alive. I have no pain, no sorrow, and no horror stories to replay in my mind over and over again. It has never been more apparent to me that we have to appreciate *today*. For tomorrow we can be drinking our morning coffee, or reading the paper, and all of a sudden it could all be gone! Jay has now joined me in the ranks of the survivors. He'll just have to get used to the word.

Journal Entry — Sunday, September 16, 2001

There is no way I'll ever be able to express the events of these last 5 days. This past Tuesday morning two planes were hijacked and flown into the World Trade Center. Both buildings have since collapsed and thousands of people have died. Another plane has crashed into the Pentagon and yet another crashed into a field in Pennsylvania. Jay was in Monte Carlo when all this happened. He finally made it home last night. Everyone in his immediate department made it out safely, but he's going to know some people from the other tower.

I am physically and emotionally drained and I have no idea how those who've lost someone are even able to cope. It frightens me to my core. I can't believe this can be happening to our country. It will change the way we live forever. I am in shock!

The 2001 Avon Breast Cancer 3-Day Walk

After the events of 9/11, the 2001 Avon 3-Day was rescheduled, from its original September date to late October, to give our country time to begin its long healing process. I agonized over postponing my mastectomy so that I could participate for the second time. My surgeon's office was understanding of my plight and worked hard to accommodate me so that I could experience this positive event once again.

Along with many of the friends I'd met at the 2000 walk, we were joined this year by a number of "first-timers." The two groups became one, and we formed a team for the event. We called ourselves the LILACs (Long Island Ladies Against Cancer). Clad in red, white and blue team uniforms and hats designed by one of our teammates, we presented ourselves as a united front against this deadly disease. We traveled in a pack throughout the three days and laughed and cried together as we helped one another take the next step when we were ready to quit.

The tone of the walk was vastly different from the previous year, however. Many of the walkers had known someone who was lost during the terrorist attack, so it became not only a walk for breast cancer but also an event for our country as a whole. It was much more solemn than the 2000 event, and while there were still cheers for all of the walkers, I was pleased to note that we weren't being heralded as "heroes" as we were the previous year. Everyone knew that the real heroes were still being discovered as more and more stories about the selfless acts of 9/11 were brought to light.

Our mission was still very important, to be sure. But those on the 2001 Avon Breast Cancer 3-Day were walking to honor all of those who lost their lives on 9/11 as well. As a breast cancer survivor, I was more than happy to relinquish last year's "hero" status, knowing that thousands of Americans were facing battles far greater than my battle with breast cancer. My cancer was just a bump in the road of my life, and I was deeply moved by all those who came out to join us in the walk against breast cancer when there were so many more pressing issues facing our country at the time. For the second year in a row I considered myself privileged to be a part of this astonishing event.

Back to Business

Now, with the second wonderful 3-Day behind me, it was back to the business at hand. I still needed to make informed decisions about my health. Ultimately, I decided to have the sentinel node procedure done along with the mastectomy. And after doing some research, although I felt rather confident about the safety of silicone implants, I decided to stick with the saline that I already had. I knew myself well enough to know that if I were to have silicone implants I would worry that any ache or pain might be caused by leaking silicone. It was a very personal decision, arrived at only after many hours of research and introspection.

I had my second mastectomy in early November 2001. Everything went smoothly and as planned, and I came home the next day. As we had hoped, the breast tissue was benign. Luckily, my surgeon was able to take the sentinel node without making another painful incision. The plastic surgeon was able to insert the "final" implant during this surgery, avoiding the weekly fill-ups of the tissue expander.

Journal Entry — Thursday, November 8, 2001
I went in last Friday for the prophylactic mastectomy. Everything went well, although I was sick overnight due to the anesthesia. I had one pain shot in the hospital and haven't even had to take any pain medication since. Last night I had a tough time with all the pulling, swelling, tightening, etc., but I can't really call

it pain. I got the drains out today and that seems to really help a lot. It was beginning to really hurt.

Today was my first real day out. I went to Brian's school for his open house — just an hour. By the time I got home I was pooped. I guess I'm not as "back to normal" as I think I am. I can't wait to get back into the swing of things. Emotionally I feel very good.

My recovery went smoothly. Since my plastic surgeon was able to insert the implant at the time of surgery, I had to go under the knife only one more time. I allowed myself ample time to heal and took a small break from the unceasing events of the last several years before scheduling the last step of my reconstruction.

I decided to complete the reconstruction process in spring 2002. It was my ninth surgery in four years; to say I was tired of it is an understatement. Given that this was just a cosmetic procedure and not life-threatening, Jay and I were almost giddy as we waited in the pre-op area prior to my going into the operating room.

My surgeon stopped by to see me before surgery. He rattled off the usual questions and explained the procedure one more time. Then he took out his marker and started marking where he would cut. I was accustomed to this procedure from my other breast reconstruction, but this time he took a different approach.

Since he was reconstructing the nipple and wanted to be sure it was symmetrical with the other breast, he began by measuring my existing nipple. Then, using those dimensions, he cut out a kind of "pasty" from a piece of paper. He then proceeded to ask for Jay's input as he moved the pasty around my newer breast until he found the correct spot. Imagine my humiliation as I sat naked from the waist up while my doctor and my husband conferred about where he should position my nipple! *"A little to the left." "Now up a bit." "No, no, move it a tad to the right." "Okay, perfect."*

If ever there was a time for a sense of humor, this was it! Jay and I could barely contain our laughter as this absurd situation unfolded. Finally, happy with their mutual decision, my doctor left the room and

I put my robe back on. Moments later, just as we were beginning to let down our guard, he returned, opened up my robe once more and put his initials on my breast. "New procedure" he would say. "They're making us put our initials on the side we're operating on; it seems there have been mistakes in the past." That was the straw that broke the camel's back! Neither of us could contain ourselves as we erupted into hysterical laughter. I felt like a groupie at a rock concert.

A minute later the nurse appeared to take me to the operating room. Jay kissed me goodbye and told me he loved me and would be there when I awoke. I was wheeled into the operating room with a smile on my face. This was the end of a long, hard road and I had my best friend by my side. Throughout all the surgeries and all the changes my body had gone through in the last three years, Jay's love and support had never wavered. If he was frightened or uncertain, he'd never let it show. There was never a time, not even once, when he made me feel unattractive! What more could I ask for?

The surgery went as planned, and my recuperation proceeded smoothly. I was thrilled to finally have two matching breasts and couldn't wait to see the final result. After all the turmoil of the past few years this was going to be my consolation prize. I had delusions of emerging with the body of a swimsuit model! *What in the world was I thinking?*

Given all the body image issues I'd had since my first mastectomy, it was especially disappointing that the final outcome was not what I had imagined. This was the last surgery I would be having on my breasts — the symbol that my breast cancer was now in my past. It was also my last chance to finally return to being a "normal" woman with two matching breasts. Sadly, that wasn't the case.

It is very difficult to achieve perfect symmetry when reconstructing with implants. In my case, the skin of one breast stretched more than the other, and the incisions were not exactly the same. Furthermore, the muscle and surrounding tissues on each side accepted the implant differently, thus arriving at a less-than-perfect result, to say the least!

Journal Entry — Monday, March 11, 2002

I had my surgery on March 7th and I came through it just fine. I feel great today — almost back to normal, except for this surgical bra, which is chafing me in some spots. My breasts are not even either — one is lower than the other. I'm trying not to get too upset since there's probably still some swelling, and with the right nipple still bandaged it's hard to see the final result. It really, really makes me mad, though. I held out so much hope for this surgery!

I was absolutely certain I had made the right decision, and I have no regrets. But I was very disheartened about the way I looked and had to work through a whole new set of insecurities. Some days are good days, and some are bad. It's all in my attitude.

On a bad day I scrutinize my body in the mirror and agonize over the asymmetry, the scarring, and the fact that my breasts have gone from a source of sexual stimulation and pleasure to something of a science experiment. It irritates me that my life has been defined by my breasts. First by my longing for them to develop, closely followed by my desire to have them *stop* developing, and finally by their attempt to kill me!

On a bad day I get angry when I try on clothes that I can't wear because they are too low cut or so clingy that it is obvious that what I refer to as breasts are simply sacks of saline water surgically implanted into my chest wall. I've spent many hours in department store fitting rooms close to tears and wanting to scream because my body looks like a mannequin, with rock-hard breasts standing at attention while the rest of my body moves in normal motion.

More important than the physical aspect is the emotional side of removing my breasts. I was fearful that Jay and I would never be able to achieve the closeness and level of intimacy we enjoyed in the past. He says it doesn't matter to him. I don't believe him...not a bit. But I think Jay knows that's what I need to hear and I love him all the more for saying it.

Most of my days, however, are good days. On those days I'm grateful that I can go braless and wear halter tops and spaghetti strap dresses for the first time in my life. When I try on clothes on a *good* day, I'm thrilled that my rock-hard, stand-at-attention breasts make my whole body look fit and create a nice curve between my neck and my waistline. I'll never again have to worry about underwire support bras or saggy breasts...even when I'm 50, or 60, or 70. Come to think of it, in trading my natural breasts for those "sacks of saline water" I now actually *believe* I may live into my 50s, 60s or even 70s! In the larger scheme of things, it was a very small price to pay for a longer, healthier life.

So now, with all this behind me, as far as I was concerned there was nothing left to take. I had removed not only my cancerous breast but my healthy breast and ovaries as well. My lymph nodes were tested and all came back negative! I had completed six months of chemotherapy and was three years into my five-year regimen of tamoxifen. Now I was well on my way to putting this all behind me once and for all. Cancer was now officially a thing of my past.

Not so for the rest of my family.

Part IV

Learning to Live
with
My Heritage

Tuna Sandwiches with Dad

Obviously being of a different lineage, Dad was the only person in my nuclear family who didn't have to worry about our genetic predisposition. So when he didn't feel well in the spring of 2002, although we were concerned, none of us had cancer on our minds. We all believed that his discomfort and shortness of breath were due to the added weight he'd packed on over the years.

When he finally decided to undergo surgery on his arthritic knees, Dad thought that he would be able to resume some activities and lose the added pounds. But after seeing the doctor for a pre-surgical workup, dreams of a healthier, pain-free lifestyle were shattered. Dad was diagnosed with emphysema, congestive heart failure, arthritis and anemia. Needless to say, his knee surgery was put on hold.

In addition, a routine chest X-ray uncovered a "spot" on the lining of his lung that they needed to biopsy. *Biopsy* ... they wanted him to have a *biopsy*. How I detested that word! It never yielded a good result when performed on anyone in my family.

Cancer, the word that had become synonymous with the Fraine family, would now be used on a Tropea. Dad was diagnosed with lung cancer on May 10, 2002, the day before his 71st birthday and nineteen years after my mother lost her battle to the same disease. He was the eighth member of my family to hear the terrifying words "You have cancer." Would any of us have the strength to go down this road again?

Journal Entry — Monday, May 20, 2002

Sometimes when things are going well I begin to get nervous that things are going to blow up. Well, it's safe to say that they blew up big time. Dad's biopsy came back positive. He was diagnosed with cancer in the lining of his lung. The doctor basically gave us no hope and said it was very fast growing.

It was such a horrible day. I feel like I am thrust right back into nearly 4 years ago, when I was diagnosed. Dad was admitted to the hospital to put a drain in his lung to help him breathe. It was very painful and he seems to be pretty depressed.

Now the tables had turned. Dad had always been worried about us. He'd waited nervously with Jay through every single one of my surgeries, leaving only after he was able to speak to me when I awoke. Once, while he was waiting outside the curtain as I undressed for a surgical procedure, I overheard him tell Jay that he wished it was happening to him instead of me — that he had lived his life already and would gladly accept the disease if it would rid me of it! What undeniable pain cancer had caused in his life. He watched his wife wither away from it, one daughter battle it, and another daughter undergo major surgery in a desperate attempt to thwart it. Now he was facing a fight of his own. Would this cancer ever let up?

The next weeks and months would have us running around finding the proper doctors and procedures that would be best for Dad. Ultimately, it was determined that my dad's lung cancer was a direct result of the asbestos he had been exposed to in various jobs held many years earlier. His cancer was considered inoperable, and chemotherapy was suggested.

My sisters and I sprang into action to be there for Dad as best we could. Once a plan of attack was laid out, Dad took himself to many of his own appointments. But when it came to chemotherapy or any new consultations, we attempted to accompany him.

Journal Entry — Tuesday, June 11, 2002

More changes. The first doctor we saw last week doesn't take Dad's insurance. What a frustrating, wasted day that was! Today we found another oncologist that we really like. Dad is scheduled to start chemo next week. This week he has all his scans — bone, chest, brain, etc.

I took him for his bone scan yesterday, so he and I spent the whole day together. He seems pretty depressed, although he won't admit it. I feel so bad and so helpless. Hopefully, when he starts the chemo it will shrink the tumor enough to give him some relief. This whole thing is so terribly sad. It's frightening how comfortable and familiar it is to me to be back in this "cancer place."

With my father living about 20 minutes west of me and his doctor being halfway between our two homes, there was a lot of driving involved on the days I took him to chemo. Add to that dealing with the lunatics on the Long Island Expressway. Dad would curse at the other drivers while telling me which lane I should be in . . . to speed up . . . or slow down . . . or pass this one or that one. Those were stressful days.

By the time his two-hour chemotherapy appointment was over, Dad would be tired and hungry. Food was a very important part of my father's life, so it was with great pleasure that he noticed a sign on the window of a delicatessen near his oncologist's office. *Two tuna sandwiches and two sodas for* $5.99.

Whenever one of us took Dad for chemo, he would insist on stopping at the deli for sandwiches on the way home. It was exasperating at first — I usually wasn't hungry, and I knew it would make me have to rush home afterward to beat the school bus. As time passed, however, I came to really enjoy our tuna sandwiches.

There is something about sharing a meal with another person, even a meal as simple as a tuna sandwich, which requires you to communicate. When there is nothing else going on except two people sitting

down to eat, you simply have to converse. We would take the sandwiches back to Dad's house and eat there.

Happy to be home after his treatment, Dad would first make himself comfortable. Next, he would take out the Italian dressing and add a
little to his sandwich. Then he'd sit down to eat, whether or not I was ready
to join him. Being a good host was never one of Dad's strong points.

I would watch as Dad devoured his lunch, all the while telling me
that he isn't really hungry, doesn't really eat that much, and has absolutely no idea how he had managed to pack 215 pounds onto his 5-foot
6-inch frame. Then he would make himself a cup of coffee and gobble
down one or two Stella D'Oro anisette toast cookies, all the while slurp-
ing, belching, and blowing his nose. I could practically hear my mother:
"Ooh Fah, Pete! Must you do that at the table?!"

Usually we talked about mundane things — maybe what I was making for dinner that night or when Jay's next business trip would be. I
would ask about his sister, my Aunt Marie, and her family. Occasionally
we would stumble upon a memory or funny story from when Mom
was alive. Sometimes he'd ask me to look over some paperwork — his
will or bank statement — and then it would be time to leave. Dad would
thank me profusely, slobber a kiss on my cheek, and I'd be out the door.

While there were seldom any heartwarming conversations and no
eloquent words of wisdom being passed from father to daughter, I still
found myself feeling good for the rest of the day. For the first time in
my life I could spend time with Dad and feel comfortable just chatting.
Perhaps it was because I also knew the feeling of sitting in a chemotherapy chair with a needle in my arm, uncertain of my future. Or
maybe it was because we were no longer just parent and child, but also
comrades reluctantly thrust into the group society has labeled "cancer
patients." Quite likely, though, it was simply because I had finally grown
up enough to see my father for the good man that he is, complete with
atrocious table manners and less than perfect communication skills. My
father is a wonderful, hardworking, honest, caring and loving man. I
am so glad that I finally had the chance to realize it. I'm sure I will never
enjoy another tuna sandwich as much as the ones I enjoyed with Dad.

Five years and several family vacations later, my dad's cancer is in remission. Chemotherapy has shrunk his tumor substantially. Having seen as much cancer as my family has seen, we are all realistic enough to know that it will probably not disappear completely. Still, we are delighted with his progress and thrilled to have been able to spend quality family time together.

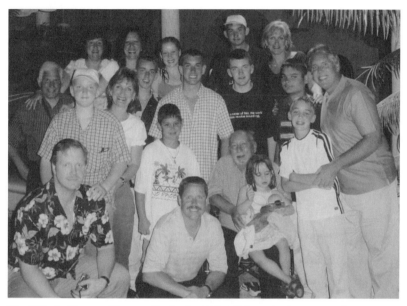

The Whole Tropea Clan — Barbados 2004. Taken during one of our many family vacations. Top row, left to right: Linda, Carol, Carissa, Albert, Laura. Middle row: Al, Brian, me, Stephen, Michael, Matthew, Christopher, Jim. Bottom row: Jay (kneeling), Nicky, George (kneeling), Dad, Alana (on lap), Andrew.

Mary's Story

When I received the news that my cousin Mary was diagnosed with breast cancer in the winter of 2003, I was very distressed, although not completely surprised. Mary is Patty's sister, another one of Uncle Bob's daughters. It seemed as if every time we were about to put a cancer behind us, someone else was diagnosed. Mary was the ninth family member.

She was 41 at her diagnosis, married with two school-age daughters. Though we lived nearly two hours away from one another, I called or e-mailed her often and gave her whatever support I could.

Journal Entry — Saturday, March 15, 2003
The sadness and despair that so many people must face totally overwhelms me at times. Mary has now been diagnosed with breast cancer. We've spoken several times already and she seems to be alright with it all. Her surgery was March 13th and she is recovering well. No word on lymph node involvement or staging yet.

It's funny, but since my own diagnosis I just assume now that people with breast cancer are going to be fine. I guess that's a really good thing, but I certainly hope I am not wrong this time.

Mary underwent a mastectomy with reconstruction and chemotherapy. After all her treatments were completed and her hair was starting to grow back in, she and her family decided to move to Florida to start a new, simpler life. Her husband had a new job and her girls were excited about starting anew. Sadly, that's when she was diagnosed with a metastasis, forcing her family to put its plans on hold.

Journal Entry — Friday, February 6, 2004
I just got word that Mary's cancer spread. My heart is breaking for her. It's just such a nightmare and so incredibly sad ... and unfair. I try to understand and have faith, but it's so very hard at times. I pray so hard for them every night.

This cancer just doesn't let up. It keeps striking and killing everyone. I can't stand it anymore!

True to the memory of the generation that came before us, Mary waged the war against her cancer privately, exhibiting grace and dignity, with her husband, John, and their daughters by her side. She bravely faced more chemotherapy treatments and the distressing loss of her hair again as she coped the best she could.

I admired her bravery when she told me, "I don't think it's my time to go yet." Her kids were so young; they still needed her. Mary was filled with hope that the treatments would keep her cancer under control so that she could continue to live her life and raise her daughters.

Sadly, *hope* cannot cure cancer . . . *nothing* can cure cancer. No one knows that better than the members of my family. Mary lost her battle on May 26, 2005.

Tears blur my vision and sting my eyes as I write this. The pain is so fresh and raw; time has not yet had a chance to dull the ache. I had hoped that Mary's tale would have a happy ending and that my generation would outsmart the cancer. I thought that we had found the key to dodge the deadly disease before it had the chance to kill any of us. Sure, it struck Patty, Mary and me, but it hadn't killed us. Until now. Mary was 43 years old, the youngest member of my family to succumb to breast cancer.

I'm not sure how Mary's death will affect my day-to-day life. Months, even years, would go by without our seeing one another. Like many families, our individual lives and distance kept us apart. Still, I knew she was there living her life — working, driving her kids to activities, helping with homework — the mundane things that make up everyday existence.

After her diagnosis, we spoke or e-mailed one another more often than in the past. Although our lives were very different, we still had a common bond. She was the daughter of my mother's brother — she was my cousin. We spent our childhood holidays together: ate the same foods, laughed at the same stories, and shared the same grandparents. We mourned together when we each lost our parents. We were family.

What do you tell children when they lose their mother when they are so young? Megan and Melissa are 9 and 11 years old. What can we tell them to give them some peace and understanding?

I am reminded of a sermon I once heard at a funeral. It was a story about a young boy questioning his teacher about a book he was reading. The child was concerned because much of the book was written at a level he couldn't quite grasp yet. The teacher told the child to dog-ear the pages he didn't yet fully comprehend, until he was old enough to understand.

The celebrant suggested that we should treat death like the book the young boy was reading. Until we have the capacity to understand it, we should just dog-ear the pages in anticipation of the day when we will fully appreciate its meaning. Perhaps Mary's daughters can dog-ear the pages of questions in their hearts about their mother's untimely death until maturity and the passage of time allows them to make their peace with it.

Mary will continue to be there for her children because she will live in their hearts for the rest of their lives. Her physical being is gone, but signs of her will be in their every breath, as she will always be a part of them. She is at peace with her mother, her father, her uncle and aunts, and they now hold all the secrets that we have yet to discover. Mary's strength will live on in her daughters, just as my mother's strength is in my fingertips as I type this passage.

Revisiting the "Cancer Place"

Ever since my diagnosis I have been seeing my doctors regularly. Every six months I see my oncologist for a blood workup and examination. I visit my gynecologist once a year and my breast surgeon every six months. I try to space out my appointments so that no more than two or three months transpire without my being examined by someone in the medical profession. This process usually gives me peace of mind, knowing that any abnormalities would be picked up at an early stage. However, terror replaced common sense when my breast surgeon suggested another biopsy in March 2004.

Though I no longer have my natural breasts, my breast surgeon still gives me breast exams. In addition to checking for abnormalities in the little remaining breast tissue, she thoroughly examines the lymph nodes under my arms. For several months she had been "watching" an enlarged lymph node under my left arm (the cancer side). Since it didn't appear to be shrinking, she wanted to biopsy it to be sure it was not cancer. Though a very simple procedure, this would be my tenth surgery in six years. More importantly, after six months of chemotherapy, five years of tamoxifen, and removal of my healthy ovaries and breast, I certainly felt that there was nothing further I could do to rid my body of this cancer. The prospect of having to face it again was debilitating.

Journal Entry — Sunday, March 21, 2004

I saw the doctor on Tuesday. We've been watching a lymph node under my left arm for 6 months now. In December it seemed to be shrinking, but now it is enlarged again. I'm going in for a biopsy tomorrow. They'll do a frozen section while I am on the table. If it's positive, they'll do a full axillary node dissection to see if it spread. I'll know as soon as I wake up if it's bad, but I won't know for certain if it's good until they send it out for further evaluation. Every time I think of it I get sick to my stomach. I knew this was how my life was going to be, with one scare after another, but I just wasn't ready for this right now. It's

only been 2 years since my last surgery. I am just not ready to go back to this
cancer place! I want to get this all over with so I can move on with my life.

After having these few days to digest it all, I know that if it is cancer, I'll
simply have to deal with it again. I just really, really don't want to, and I am very
frightened right now. Hopefully I'll be writing in here tomorrow to say that
things are going well and that it was benign. Please, please, please . . . let it be
benign!

As we had done so often in the past, Jay and I drove to the day-op
center in relative silence the morning of the biopsy. There were really
no words to express what was in our hearts as we braced ourselves for
the possibility of dealing with another malignancy, after all the precau-
tions we had taken. Dad met us there, hobbling in with his cane and
leaving his oxygen tank in the car in case of an emergency. It was ironic
that he was now back in the role of caregiver, having recently completed his own chemotherapy. We joked that it was far better being the
one in the waiting room than the one being wheeled in for surgery.

The swollen lymph node was removed on a Tuesday, in a short procedure that took less than an hour. I was sedated without general anesthesia, so I was alert when I awoke. The initial biopsy results were benign, although I still had to await further testing. The three of us went to
lunch afterward. We were all relieved, though cautiously so.

Journal Entry — Tuesday, March 23, 2004
So far, so good. The frozen section was benign. I need to wait for the final results
so I am still a little nervous.

The week moved on in slow motion as we anxiously awaited the
final results. My mind drifted back to another time — the time before
cancer loomed so ominously around me, affecting my every decision.
Back to a time when life was simpler . . . and happier . . . and more
joyous. Or was it? Was life really better before the cancer?

I became very introspective, questioning my life's decisions, as if
this was my last chance to right any wrongs. If I die, *would my life have been*

worthwhile? Am I happy? Did Jay and I take advantage of our time together? Do my children know how much joy they have brought into my life and how proud I am of them? Do I have any regrets?

No matter how hard I tried, I couldn't turn off the voice inside my head. Blissfully, I came to realize that there was almost nothing in my life that I would change. Though my life is not perfect, I was truly happy and contented. I surely didn't want to die, but if cancer was going to kill me this time, I had no regrets.

The call finally came on Friday: the lymph node was benign! Benign! Oh, how I have come to love that word!

Linda Takes a Stand

With Mary's heartbreaking death still fresh in our minds, Linda was ready to proceed with the plans she had been exploring for months. Being a BRCA2 mutation carrier, she had always known the day would come when she would consider having a bilateral prophylactic mastectomy. Having undergone a biopsy three months earlier, which fortunately was benign, Linda decided to take matters into her own hands and remove the very objects that have taunted and threatened so many of our family members. She was not going to be another victim!

After exploring her options for reconstruction, Linda decided on saline implants and found a plastic surgeon who took a different approach than mine did. Linda's surgeon inserted a "permanent expander" at the time of her mastectomy, eliminating the need for three separate surgeries to complete the process. Her surgery was in June 2005 and she was home from the hospital after a brief two-night stay.

Regrettably, Linda has had to deal with an array of benign complications regarding the reconstruction. After several corrective procedures failed to remedy the situation, she ultimately decided to have the implants removed and TRAM flap surgery performed. In spite of her unfortunate circumstances, Linda stands by her decision and more importantly, she can now rest easy knowing that her breast cancer risk has been reduced by 90 percent.

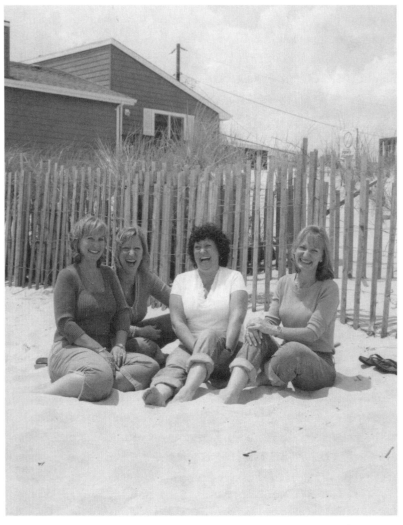

The Four Tropea Girls — July 2006. All grown up. (Courtesy of David A. Land. This photo first appeared in *Family Circle* magazine.)

Part V

The Rest
of
My Life

The Rest of My Life

I can barely remember a time when cancer wasn't part of my life. Starting back in the seventies during my teenage years, it haunted, taunted, scorned, and defied me until it became literally a part of my very being. It has threatened to take away everything I love and hold dear and has caused me to waste far too much valuable time mourning my losses and feeling sorry for myself, instead of counting my blessings. It has taken lives, shattered dreams, and left my family vulnerable and afraid — but it *did not win*. Cancer cannot take our spirit, and it cannot take our soul — and therefore it will never, ever win.

I must admit that I do think about death quite often, but I don't allow it to debilitate me. It helps me realize how fragile life is. I appreciate every day that I have, and I value the time spent with those I love.

Most of the time I can keep things in perspective, although there are still those occasions — if someone's cancer has spread or I feel an unusual pain — when that all-too-familiar panic attempts to takes over. When that happens, I reflect on all I have done to rid my body of this horrific disease . . . the mastectomies, the oophorectomy, the chemo, the tamoxifen . . . and I begin to calm down. Then I force myself to do the things that make me feel alive and keep my mind and body active. I'll work out, take a walk, or write in my journal. And I pray. Not that I won't get cancer again . . . well, *maybe* I do pray that I won't get cancer again, but I pray that if I do, I'll have the strength to get through it once more.

Years have passed since Uncle Bob, Mom, Uncle Nicky and Aunt Mary Jane lost their lives to cancer. Since then there has been tremendous progress in diagnosis and treatment, and great strides in the area of genetic testing. Quite possibly, had they known they were genetically predisposed, my mother and her siblings would have been able to diffuse the time bomb that ticked within them. Though tragic, their experiences provided the next generation with the fortitude to continue the fight. We grew up surrounded by the disease. Our awareness was a gift borne from our parents' struggle. It better prepared us to confront the enemy, and recognize it as a battle for our lives.

We've learned to be conscientious about our exams and screenings, and courageous in our treatments — some considered drastic — all to evade the disease. We know we cannot cure cancer, but we can certainly take action to intercept it. And by my being outspoken about my family's plight, there may be other women who will now take a proactive approach to their health and well-being.

Patty and I are still healthy and vibrant — the first breast cancer survivors our family has ever known. Until we tragically lost Mary, my generation was beating cancer. Her death was a shattering blow, but it reminds us that while we've made tremendous progress, we are not out of the woods. Reluctantly we took a step backwards, and then forged ahead with even greater purpose.

Mary now joins the others whose premature deaths continue to teach us about life. In the years to come, I trust her daughters will realize their full potential by drawing on her strength and memory, as I have on my own mother's.

I don't know who I would have become had I not lost my mother so early in my life. Perhaps I would have been a better person, a wiser person. Perhaps not. I envied other women shopping for their wedding gowns with their mothers by their sides, and desperately longed for her after my children were born. I needed her encouragement when, as a brand new mother, I couldn't get Matthew to nurse, and when Brian was rushed to the hospital with a febrile seizure as an infant. Mom wasn't there to assure me that my children were developing normally; that walking and potty training will happen, and broken hearts will mend. Nevertheless, over the years the pain of her absence has been replaced with gratitude for all that I have learned from her death.

She may not have been around to teach me how to cook or sew, but she trained me for something far greater than that. My mother taught me how to live life to the fullest, and how to fight illness with dignity.

Recently a friend asked me how I was able to find my tumor, being it was so small. "I was looking for it" was my response. I was expecting it, as if I knew somehow that my mother's breast cancer was simply practice for my own. Mom prepared me well.

Over eight years have passed since the fateful telephone call that changed my life. My children are eight years older and wiser, and I have had eight more years to love them, guide them, and watch them grow into the loving, caring and wonderful young men they are today. I savor every moment I have with my family and I am deeply grateful for the time we have been able to spend together.

Matthew and Brian are very aware of my genetic status and the role that cancer has played in the lives of relatives they never met. I am proud to say that they have shown wisdom far beyond their years in the way they have supported me. They don pink ribbons during breast cancer awareness month, collect money in school, and walk for the cause. I have been blessed with two children that any parent would long for. My hope is that through further scientific research, they will never have to worry about their own possible genetic predisposition.

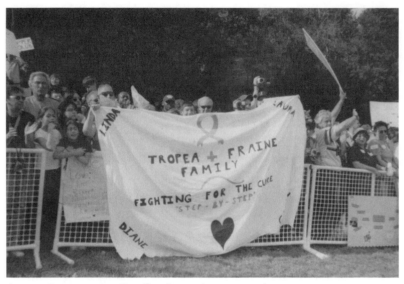

Avon 3-Day — 2000. Our families welcoming us home.

Jay and I have celebrated over 20 years of marriage so far, and anticipate a future filled with good health, love, and laughter, as we watch our boys become men. I look forward to someday welcoming daughters-in-law and grandchildren into our hearts and our home. And I pray that my children will never experience the sadness that cancer has caused their ancestors, and that the grief that befell my mother's generation will remain a distant lesson for us all.

From time to time I'll run into someone who knows of my family history and feels sorry for me, as if my life is so tragic. Quite frankly, I find it a bit ironic. While they are feeling sorry for me and my past, I have come to appreciate all it has taught me. The sickness I've experienced has left me a decidedly more enlightened person. As far as I'm concerned, I have everything — a husband and two children whom I adore, good friends and family, and a heightened awareness of what is really important in life.

After all, what constitutes a life? It is not simply the number of years you were given, but rather how you spent those years and how many lives you have touched. Though much of my family was robbed of their golden years, they left a profound and indelible mark on future generations.

I am proud to call myself my mother's daughter.

References

Brose MS, Rebbeck TR, Calzone KA, Stopfer JE, Nathanson KL, Weber BL. Cancer risk estimates for BRCA1 mutation carriers identified in a risk evaluation program. *Journal of the National Cancer Institute* 2002;94:1365–72.

Domchek SM, Garber JE. Genetic testing for breast cancer. *Principles and Practice of Oncology Updates* 2001;15:1–16.

Duffy Jr., M.D., F.A.C.S., Frederick J. DIEP/SIEA Flap Details. DIEP/SIEA Flaps in Breast reconstruction. 2005. www.dallasdiep.com/diep_flap_details.html (accessed May 21, 2006).

Duffy Jr., M.D., F.A.C.S., Frederick J. TRAM Flap Reconstruction. Dallas Breast Reconstruction. 2005. www.dallasdiep.com/tram_flap_recontstruction.html (accessed May 21, 2006). [Misspelling of "recontstruction" is necessary to access the Web page.]

Grigg Martha, Bondurant Stuart, Ernster Virginia L., Herdman Roger, editors. *Information for Women About the Safety of Silicone Breast Implants*. A report of a study by the Institute of Medicine. Copyright 2000 by the National Academy of Sciences.

Komenaka IK, Ditkoff B-A, Joseph K-A, et al. The development of interval breast malignancies in patients with BRCA mutations. *Cancer* 2004;100:2079–2085.

Miki Y, Swensen J, Shattuck-Eidens P, et al. A strong candidate for the breast and ovarian cancer susceptibility gene BRCA1. *Science* 1994;266:66–71.

National Cancer Institute. Genetic Testing for BRCA1 and BRCA2: It's Your Choice. *National Cancer Institute FactSheet.* February 6, 2002. www.cancer.gov/cancertopics/factsheet/Risk/BRCA

National Cancer Institute. Preventive Mastectomy: Questions and Answers. *National Cancer Institute FactSheet.* March 21, 2005. www.cancer.gov/cancertopics/factsheet/Therapy/preventive-mastectomy.

National Cancer Institute. Tamoxifen: Questions and Answers. *National Cancer Institute FactSheet.* May 13, 2002. www.cancer.gov/cancertopics/factsheet/Therapy/tamoxifen.

National Comprehensive Cancer Network (NCCN), American Cancer Society (ACS). *Breast Cancer Treatment Guidelines for Patients.* Version VII — August 2005.

NIH Consensus Conference. Treatment of early-stage breast cancer. *JAMA*;265:391–395.

Rebbeck TR, Friebel T, Lynch HT, et al. Bilateral prophylactic mastectomy reduces breast cancer risk in BRCA1 and BRCA2 mutation carriers: The PROSE study group. *Journal of Clinical Oncology* 2004;22:1055–1062.

Wooster R, Bignell G, Lancaster J, et al. Identification of the breast cancer susceptibility gene BRCA2. *Nature* 1995;38:789–92.

Resources

Breast Cancer Resources

Adelphi NY Statewide Breast Cancer Hotline & Support Program
1-800-877-8077
www.adelphi.edu/nysbreastcancer

American Cancer Society
1-800-ACS-2345
www.cancer.org

American Society of Plastic and Reconstructive Surgeons (ASPC)
1-888-4-PLASTIC
www.plasticsurgery.org

Cancer Care, Inc.
1-800-813-HOPE
www.cancercare.org

The Maurer Foundation for Breast Health Education
1-800-853-LEARN
www.maurerfoundation.org

National Breast Cancer Coalition (NBCC)
1-800-622-2838
www.natlbcc.org

National Cancer Institute (NCI)
1-800-4-CANCER
www.cancer.gov

National Coalition for Cancer Survivorship
1-877-622-7937
www.canceradvocacy.org

National Lymphedema Network
1-800-541-3259
www.lymphnet.org

Susan G. Komen Breast Cancer Foundation
1-800-462-9273
www.breastcancerinfo.com

Y-Me National Breast Cancer Organization
1-800-221-2141
www.yme.org

High Risk Information

**Memorial Sloan Kettering: High Risk
Special Surveillance Breast Program**
1-800-525-2225
www.mskcc.org/mskcc/html/8510.cfm

Strang High Risk Information and Registry
1-212-794-4900
www.strang.org

**Women at Risk Program —
Columbia-Presbyterian Medical Center**
1-800-543-2782
www.breastmd.org/war.html

Facing our Risk of Cancer Empowered (FORCE)
1-866-824-RISK
www.facingourrisk.com

National Society of Genetic Counselors
www.nsgc.org

Breast Cancer Walks

Making Strides Against Breast Cancer
www.cancer.org/stridesonline

Avon Walk for Breast Cancer
www.avonwalk.org

Breast Cancer 3-Day
www.the3day.org

The Susan G. Komen Race for the Cure
www.komen.org

About the Author

Diane Tropea Greene is a breast cancer survivor and an active volunteer at the Adelphi NY Statewide Breast Cancer Hotline & Support Program, located in Garden City, New York. She speaks extensively to women's groups about a variety of breast cancer issues, including the subject of genetic breast cancer and genetic testing.

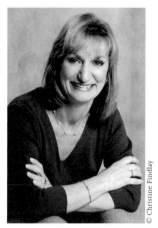

Diane Tropea Greene

She has been featured in local and national media discussing her family history with breast cancer, including *Family Circle* magazine, *Rosie* magazine and *New York Newsday*. She has also been interviewed for television news stories on ABC-TV, WPIX-TV, News-12 Long Island and WLNY-LI Cable News.

Diane was born in The Bronx and grew up in Queens Village, New York. She now resides on Long Island with her husband and two teenage boys. She welcomes visitors to her website:

www.ApronStringsBook.com